IDRC-043e

DOCTORS AND HEALERS

ALEXANDER DOROZYNSKI

Alexander Dorozynski is the author of several books and many articles, chiefly on medical and scientific subjects. He was also the founding editor and later publisher of *Médecine Mondiale,* a European newsmagazine for physicians. The views expressed in this booklet are his own. They do not necessarily represent the views of the IDRC.

Foreword

Every country has accorded major priority, at least in public statements, to the provision of health care to all the people. Very few have realized this goal. There are several reasons for this failure, including inadequate political and budgetary commitment and most importantly, lack of commitment to changing social and political structures that are basic to the improved health and well-being of all groups in any society. Another fundamental issue is the system of health care that is adapted. Developing countries, in their desire to "catch up" to the richer ones, have emulated the models of modern medicine — training of physicians, high levels of technical specialization, expensive hospitals, curative medicine. But is this model the correct one? Can governments afford this approach? Even if they could, would this be the most effective and least disruptive way of providing health care? And what would be lost to the society, in terms of existing traditional health care resources?

Clearly, innovative approaches are needed to assure that adequate basic health services are easily available to everyone, at a price that everyone, and all nations, can afford. New kinds of health workers are needed, and in large numbers. But beyond this, we need to take the primary responsibility for individual health out of the hands of the professional worker, and back to the individual. Ultimately, we are each responsible for our own health. If the "system" is not tailored to this end, the result will be dependence on high-powered technology and on highly-trained specialists. This leads to the dehumanization of the health process.

The problem then comes full circle. The rich countries are facing the dilemma of extremely costly impersonal health services. An increasing number of concerned individuals realize that fundamental changes are needed, but the problem of overcoming entrenched institutions is enormous. There is still time for the developing countries to create new models, more appropriate to their own traditions, capabilities and financial means. It may be that they have a significant advantage in not being as yet totally committed to the inappropriate systems of the richer nations.

Mr. Dorozynski has posed many of these questions, and has described a few of the new approaches being initiated. The International Development Research Centre, along with various governments and international agencies, has supported a variety of innovative programs designed to provide practical approaches to the provision of health care services, one of the most pressing problems in the world today. This provocative booklet effectively highlights the issues at stake, and will serve to stimulate discussion on this fundamental question that affects us all.

George F. Brown, Director
Population Health Sciences Division
International Development Research Centre

CONTENTS

DOCTORS

AND

HEALERS

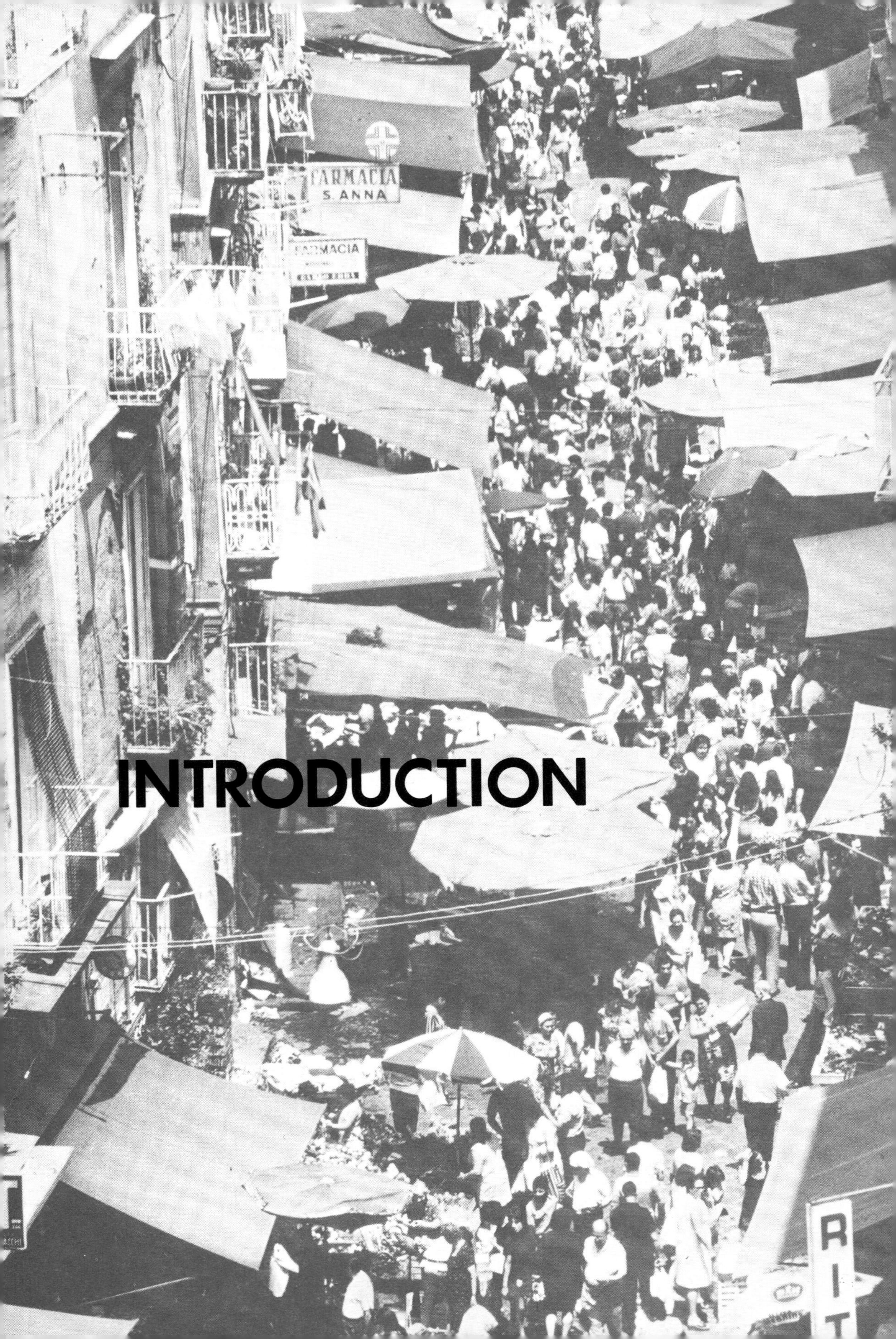

INTRODUCTION

Health is said to be a human right, that is, a condition to which everyone has a just claim. The very acceptance of the notion of human right implies that society assumes a responsibility and will give high priority to carrying it out.

Health, of course, includes a number of components such as sanitary education, adequate food and housing, good drinking water, protection against communicable diseases, access to the means of controlling one's own fertility, as well as the more directly "medical" aspects of prevention and treatment of diseases.

Obviously the right to health is not a reality to all the people of the earth. Hundreds of millions are underfed and poorly housed, and only a small percentage of the rural population of the developing countries have access to safe and adequate supplies of water. Communicable diseases are still widespread. And health care delivery — the delivery of the extraordinarily effective means of prevention and treatment known today — is non-existent in many of the developing world's rural areas.

A stereotyped approach

It is with this latter aspect — health care delivery — that this publication is concerned, because it is becoming increasingly apparent that a stereotyped approach has almost universally been adopted that hampers effective health care delivery in much of the world. The stereotype is that of the Western medical system, which prevails no matter what a country's social or economic condition, political system, or religious beliefs. Of course it is true that delivery of adequate food or housing or good water is also hampered by factors other than poverty, but the reasons for maldistribution or mismanagement are less uniform than they are with respect to health care delivery.

The text that follows is based on the observations of the author and others, but obviously certain facts have been selected or stressed because they contribute to making a point : that there is a virtual monopoly concerning health care delivery, and that the monopoly does not always serve the best interests of all people. Other methods of health care delivery can be not only more effective under certain conditions, but also much less costly than those corresponding to the pattern set by the medical establishment.

Finding one's own way

Some authors have gone further, maintaining that modern medicine has reached a point where it does not effectively treat, but instead creates disease. This viewpoint is more difficult to defend, although there is no doubt that in some highly industrialized countries there exists a form of medical and pharmacological addiction. Statistics can easily show that people who are provided with "the best medecine" do not necessarily enjoy the best health. It is not always easy for policy-makers in one country to be aware of conditions in other countries, and to benefit from the experience of others. It is always difficult to break away from an established system, surrounded and supported by its established hierarchy ; but breaking away may be necessary in order to find one's own path to progress, rather than following a path set by others, which may lead the wrong way.

This publication does not attempt to recommend one solution or another, but to show that there are many solutions to the problem of health care delivery. In this respect it corresponds to the policy the International Development Research Centre, which does not provide medical aid in the form of physicians, drugs, or the support of classical medical education, but encourages projects that tend to develop original solutions by resorting to tiers of medical workers with different skills and levels corresponding to the needs and the demand of a particular region or country ●

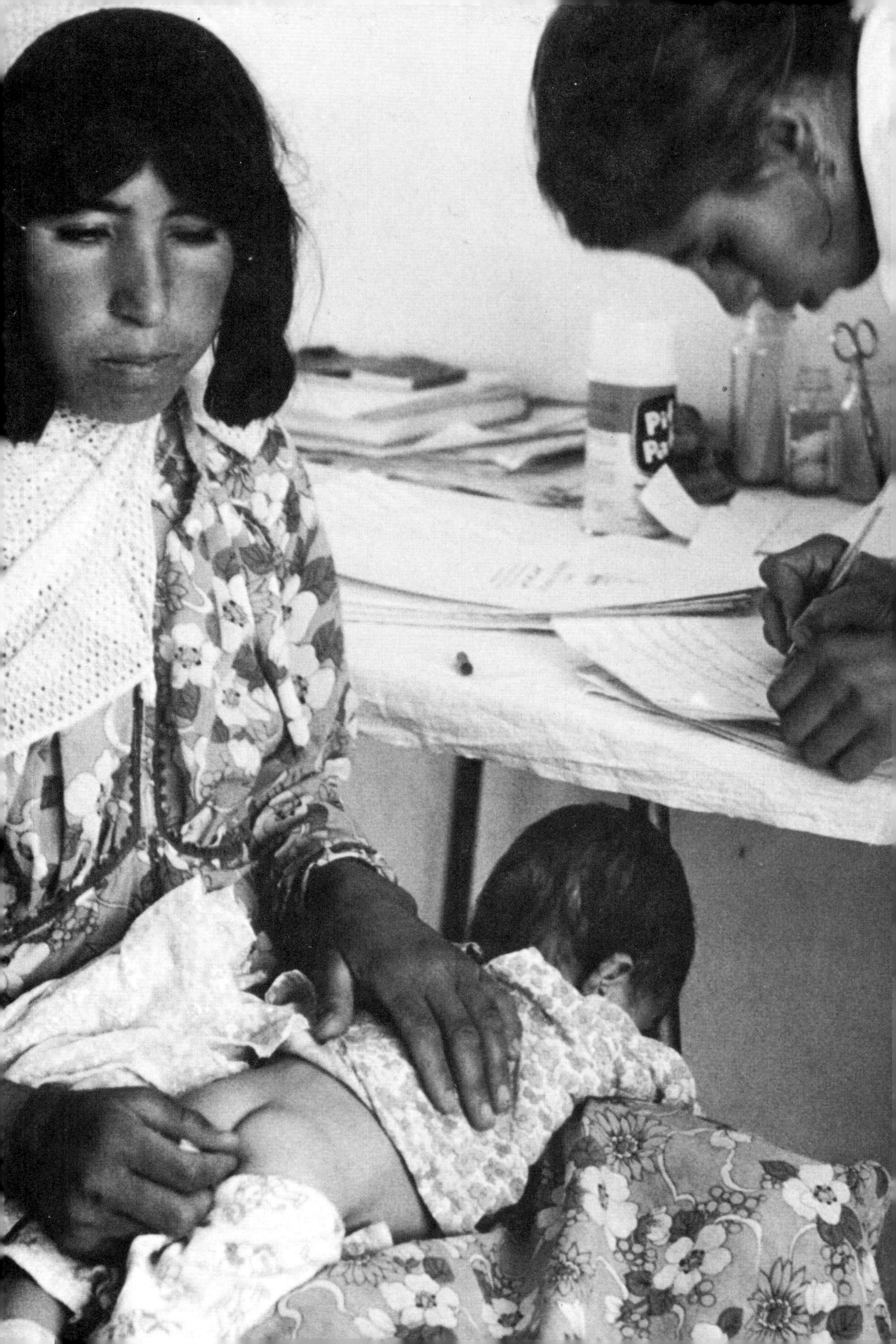

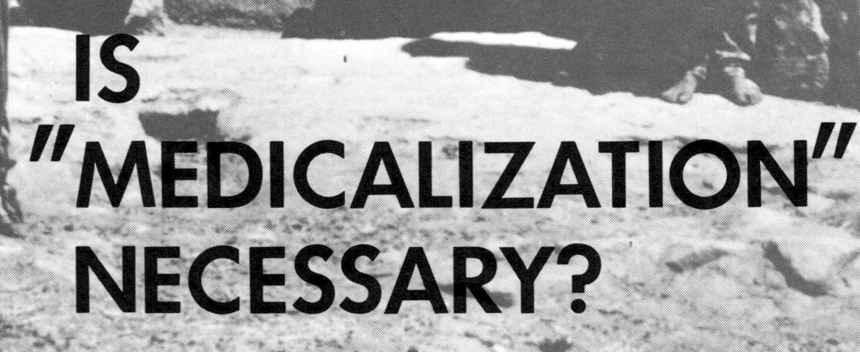

IS "MEDICALIZATION" NECESSARY?

"If I were asked to compose an epitaph on medicine throughout the 20th century, it would read : brilliant in its discoveries, superb in its technological breakthroughs, but woefully inept in its applications to those most in need. Medicine will be judged not on its vast and rapid accumulation of knowledge per se, but on its trusteeship of that knowledge. We are now experienced, and all that remains is the problem of translating what is common knowledge and routine medicine, and hence practice, to the other two-thirds of the world. The implementation gap must be closed."
Dr. N.R.E. Fendall, head,
Department of Tropical Community Medicine
University of Liverpool, U.K.

IS "MEDICALIZATION" NECESSARY ?

There are approximately 2.5 million medical doctors in the world. This represents a "medical density" of about 8 doctors for 10 000 people, or 1250 people per doctor. (China, which possesses a unique health care delivery system, is exluded from these statistics, and will be discussed in a separate section). Of course these medical doctors are not evenly spread throughout the world. Medical density varies to a great extent, from less than one doctor for 100 000 people, to one doctor for 400 people. In other words, in some places people never see a doctor at all ; in others, doctors compete among themselves for patients.

Medical density and health

A gross maldistribution becomes evident when medical density is broken down by countries or regions. In Africa as a whole, medical density is about 1.4 per 10 000 people. But in Africa as everywhere else, doctors tend to gather in large cities, so that rural populations are without any medical services except the occasional visit of a mobile team, usually carrying out an immunization program. In Asia medical density is less than 3 doctors per 10 000 people, and in Latin America, it is about 6.5. The countries with the greatest medical densities are Israel, with 25 doctors per 10 000 people, and the Soviet Union, 24.

It is difficult, however, to establish a positive correlation between medical density and health (or with life expectancy, which lends itself more easily to statistical study). Results are sometimes conflicting. Bin-Dang-Ha Doan, director of the Centre for Medical Sociology and Demography in Paris, has recently published in *World Health Statistics* a study that shows a general correlation between medical density and life expectancy. An American researcher, Charles T. Stewart, has published in *The Journal of*

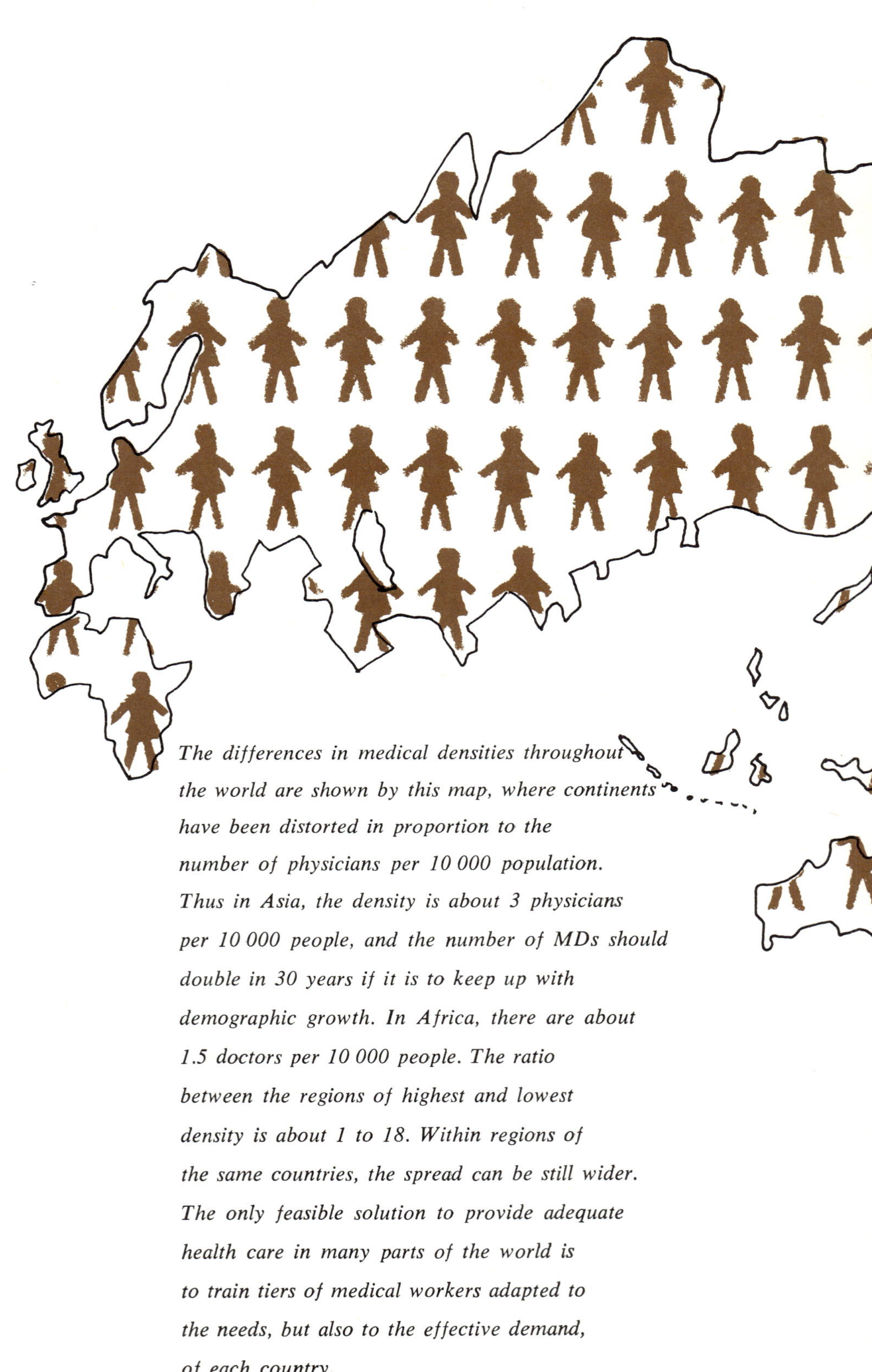

The differences in medical densities throughout the world are shown by this map, where continents have been distorted in proportion to the number of physicians per 10 000 population. Thus in Asia, the density is about 3 physicians per 10 000 people, and the number of MDs should double in 30 years if it is to keep up with demographic growth. In Africa, there are about 1.5 doctors per 10 000 people. The ratio between the regions of highest and lowest density is about 1 to 18. Within regions of the same countries, the spread can be still wider. The only feasible solution to provide adequate health care in many parts of the world is to train tiers of medical workers adapted to the needs, but also to the effective demand, of each country.

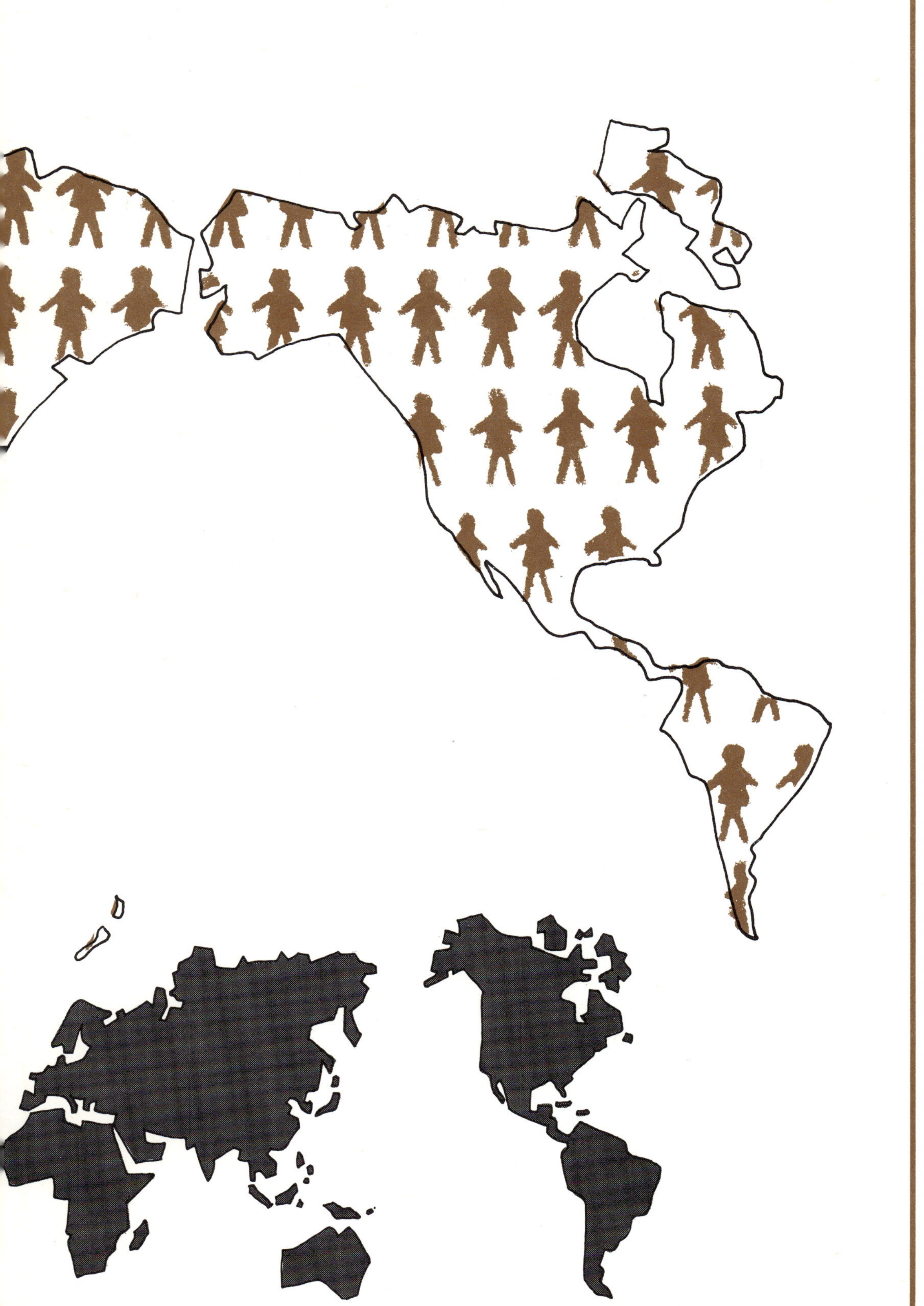

Human Resources evidence indicating that the opposite may be true. For instance, he found that the life-span is essentially the same in a number of countries where medical density varies between 4 and 16 doctors per 10 000 people.

From under to over-medication

In fact, it is easier to show that good health is related to hygiene, adequate food, good water and housing conditions than to the number of doctors in a population. This is true of industrial countries as well as developing ones. A recent study by the World Health Organization shows that in a number of industrial countries, the life expectancy of people over 60 has started declining. In most of these countries, the number of medical doctors has been steadily growing, and health expenditures increasing much more rapidly than the gross national product. But living conditions in highly industrial countries can be harmful, and a high medical density does not seem to help (perhaps because Western medicine concerns itself with individual, curative medicine, rather than with prevention through the elimination of conditions that encourage ill health). Indeed, there are indications that societies can reach a point of "over-medication" harmful to health.

The staggering cost of doctors...

Medical over-consumption, however, is the concern of relatively few. One of the major problems in the world today is how to provide the best possible health care in medically underpopulated regions, where mortality and morbidity are high.

On the surface, the answer may seem obvious : increase the number of doctors where there is a shortage. For most of the developing world, this is just not feasible within the foreseeable future. For Africa to reach Europe's medical density today would require multiplying the current number of doctors there by ten. If this goal were to be reached in 25 years – seemingly a more reasonable perspective – the number of physicians should be multiplied by 20 in order to keep up with demographic growth. The cost is staggering.

In addition, it is unlikely that there would be sufficient "effective economic demand" for the services of highly trained professionals, who might then migrate to other countries, or give up medicine to go into government, politics or business. Both these things are already happening. The medical brain drain from poor to rich countries, and the number of doctors engaged in activities other than medicine, are vivid illustrations of often futile efforts to produce in quality something very costly indeed, and for which there is no effective local demand – the Western-style medical doctor. But there are other solutions •

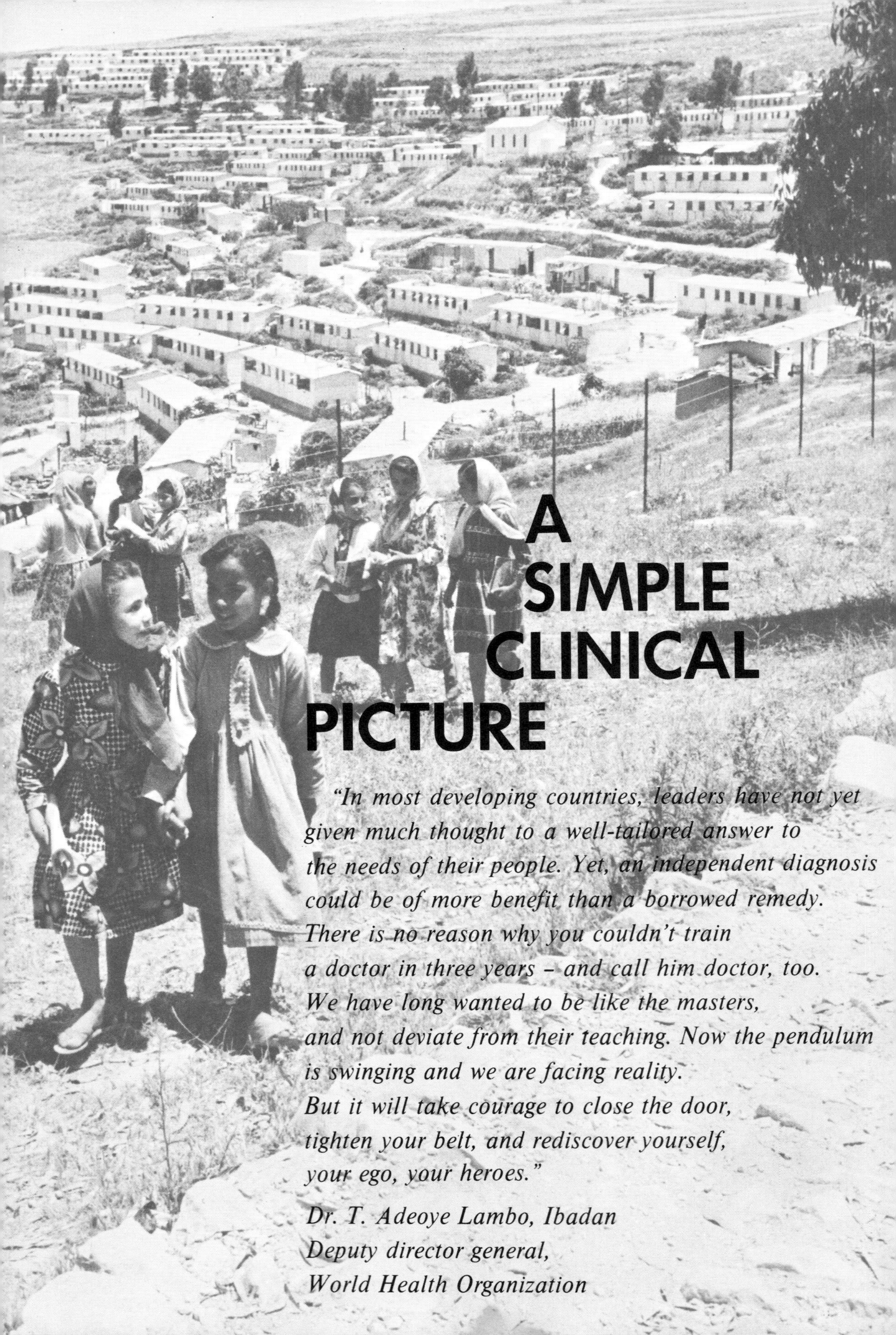

A
SIMPLE
CLINICAL
PICTURE

"In most developing countries, leaders have not yet
given much thought to a well-tailored answer to
the needs of their people. Yet, an independent diagnosis
could be of more benefit than a borrowed remedy.
There is no reason why you couldn't train
a doctor in three years – and call him doctor, too.
We have long wanted to be like the masters,
and not deviate from their teaching. Now the pendulum
is swinging and we are facing reality.
But it will take courage to close the door,
tighten your belt, and rediscover yourself,
your ego, your heroes."

Dr. T. Adeoye Lambo, Ibadan
Deputy director general,
World Health Organization

A SIMPLE CLINICAL PICTURE

World-wide statistics on morbidity and mortality are at best approximate. Their sources are often unreliable, and the overall picture may be inaccurate. The following one does not claim to be any better, as it only averages out some of the available figures in an attempt to give an idea of the problem to be solved before the theoretical right to health even comes near to being a factual right of man.

Health expenditures in the world vary between less than $1 per person per year in some of the poorest countries, to $100 and more in wealthier ones. Average life expectancy at birth ranges from 30 to 75 years. But the pattern of disease is such that nothing varies as much as the chances for a child to survive long enough to become an adult. Mortality rates for children in the developing countries are about 100 times higher than in developed countries.

Children are the first victims

A recent estimate is given *Paediatrics Priorities in the Developing World,* by Dr. David Morley. It suggests that "whereas in the developed countries each year half a million children die during the first 5 years of life, the corresponding figure for the developing worlds is 20 million ; or, expressed as deaths per year per million of under-fives, 625 in the developed countries, and 48 000 in the developing countries."

Most of these children die of preventable or easily curable diseases. Of course in an overwhelming majority of the cases there is a composite picture of malnutrition and poor sanitation, which make the child vulnerable to illnesses that might otherwise be benign. The World Health Organization, which pools statistics from all member countries, estimates that about 90 million children under five suffer from malnutrition in the world today. Of these,

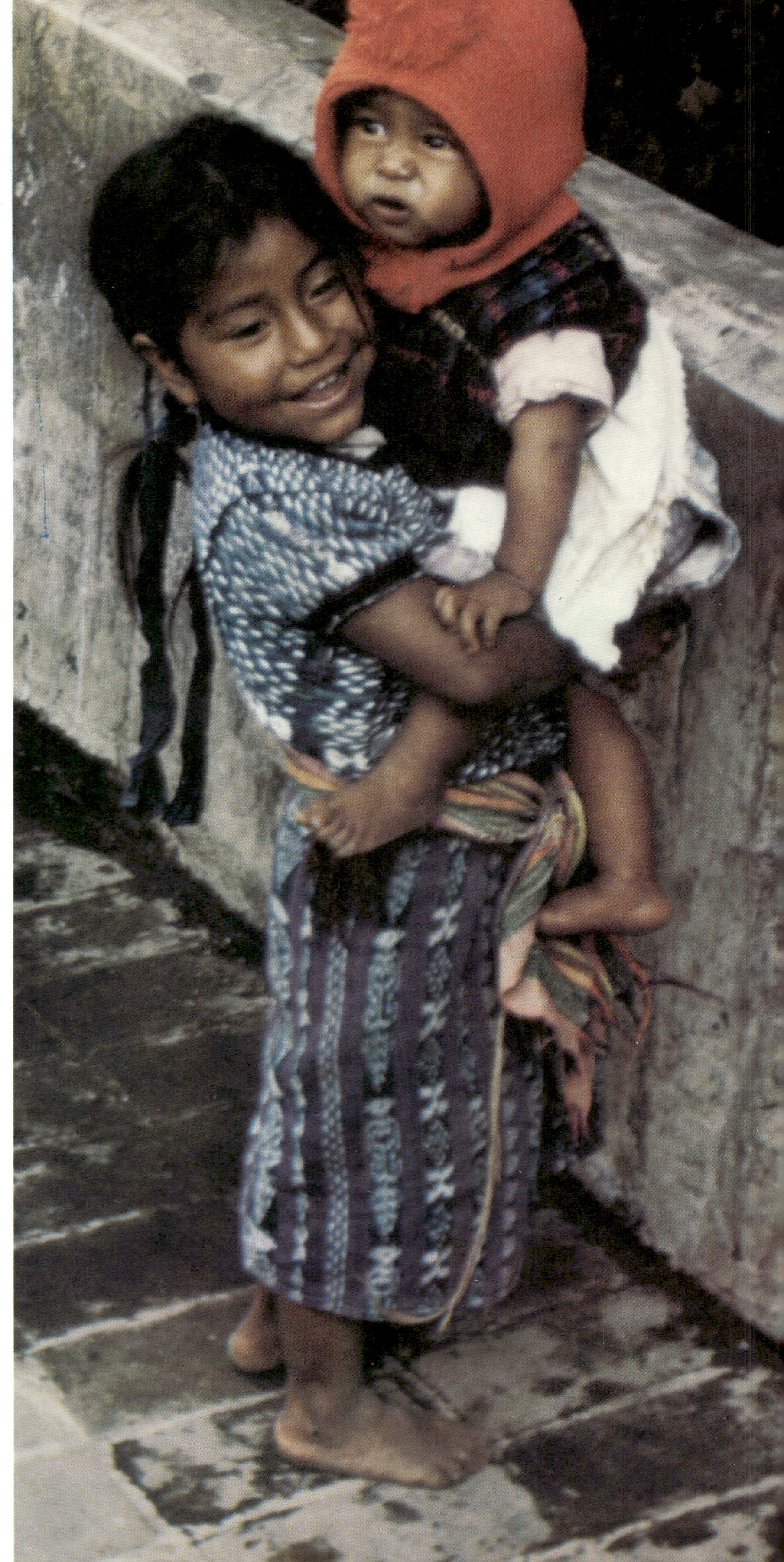

Mortality rates for children are about 100 times higher in developing countries than in developed ones. Malnutrition and infection are the principal threats to the health of these Indian children in Guatemala.

10 million are the victims of severe malnutrition. Malnutrition itself, particularly when it is the result of a shortage of protein and calories, can be lethal. But more often it is not – it opens the door to other diseases. It is estimated that children in the developing countries suffer from one type of infection or another for at least one third of their first two years of life. In some populations, measles is 400 times as lethal as in others.

The principal causes of death

The most widespread, direct cause of death is represented by respiratory infections – pneumonia, bronchitis, bronchiolitis, otitis media, croup, tonsilitis... and the common cold. Second comes diarrhoea – either the result of a gastric infection, or the reaction of the fragile, highly vascularized digestive system of the child to another insult, whether infective, toxic, even thermal. In general, between one third and two thirds of children's deaths can be attributed to combined malnutrition and infection.

Treatment can be simple

Are medical doctors, possessing a background of 20 years of education, really essential to the recognition and treatment of this disease pattern in every individual case ?

With regard to malnutrition, certainly not. Malnutrition may have many causes, from shortage of food to ignorance of the value of different types of food. Once the pattern is known, the solution is of an economical, political or educational order. Sometimes satisfactory results can be achieved by explaining that the piece of meat traditionally set aside for the working father should be given to the growing child, while the piece of sugar reserved for the child should go to the father.

The vast majority of diseases superimposed upon malnutrition are easily recognized and treated effectively with relatively inexpensive drugs. In some countries, child mortality has been radically reduced by teaching barely literate people to recognize pneumonia, and to treat it with simple means – i.e., sulfonamides, eventually backed-up with antibiotics. Likewise, in the treatment of diarrhoea,

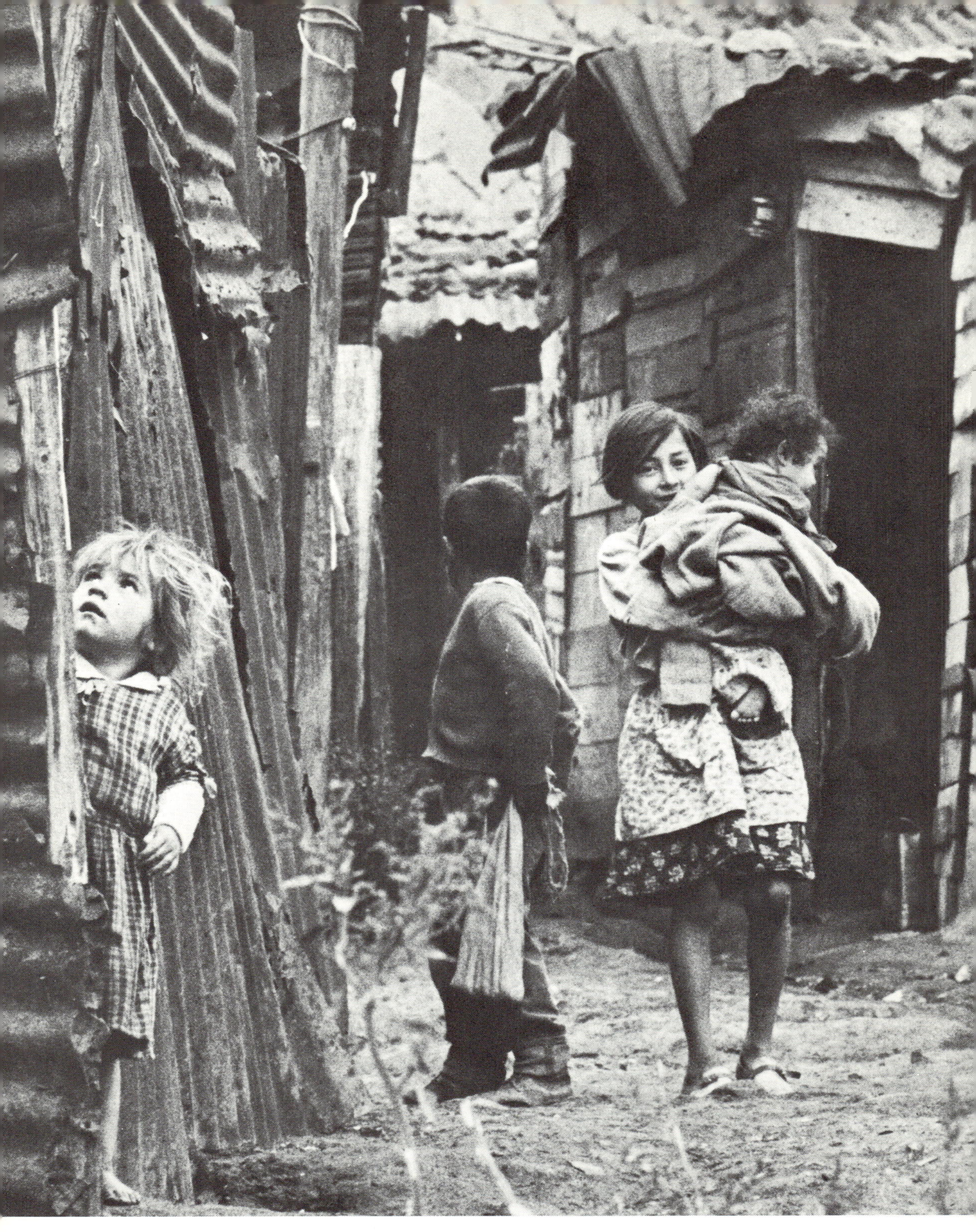

Poor housing and sanitation contribute
to spreading infection . These children
in one of the slums in Santiago, Chile,
are to benefit from a housing program.

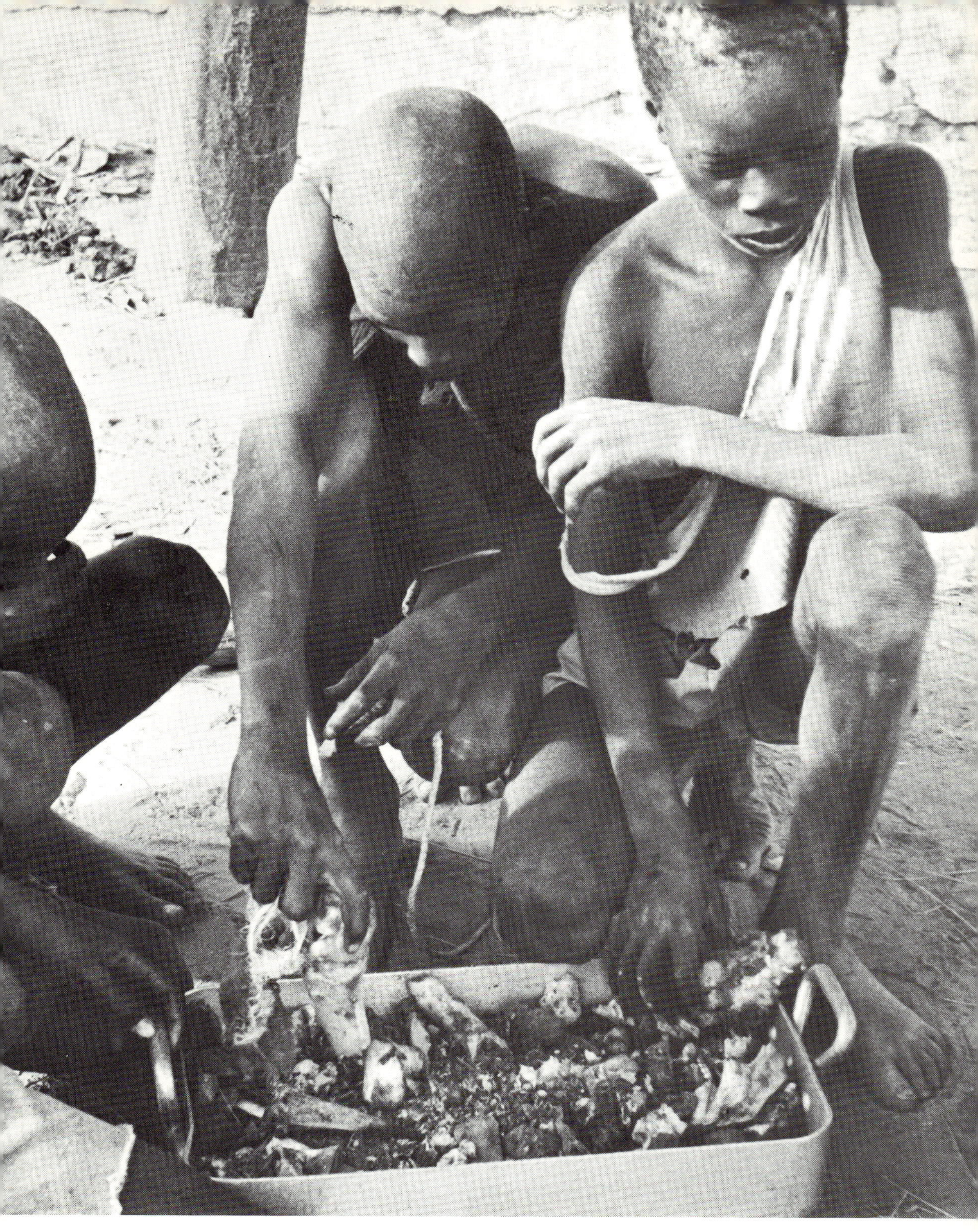

It is estimated that 90 million children
under five suffer from malnutrition.
These boys, in Mauritania, chew
bones in an "emergency kitchen."

(following page) Children in a day care
centre in Pakistan. The centre is part
of a college where students
are trained in welfare education.

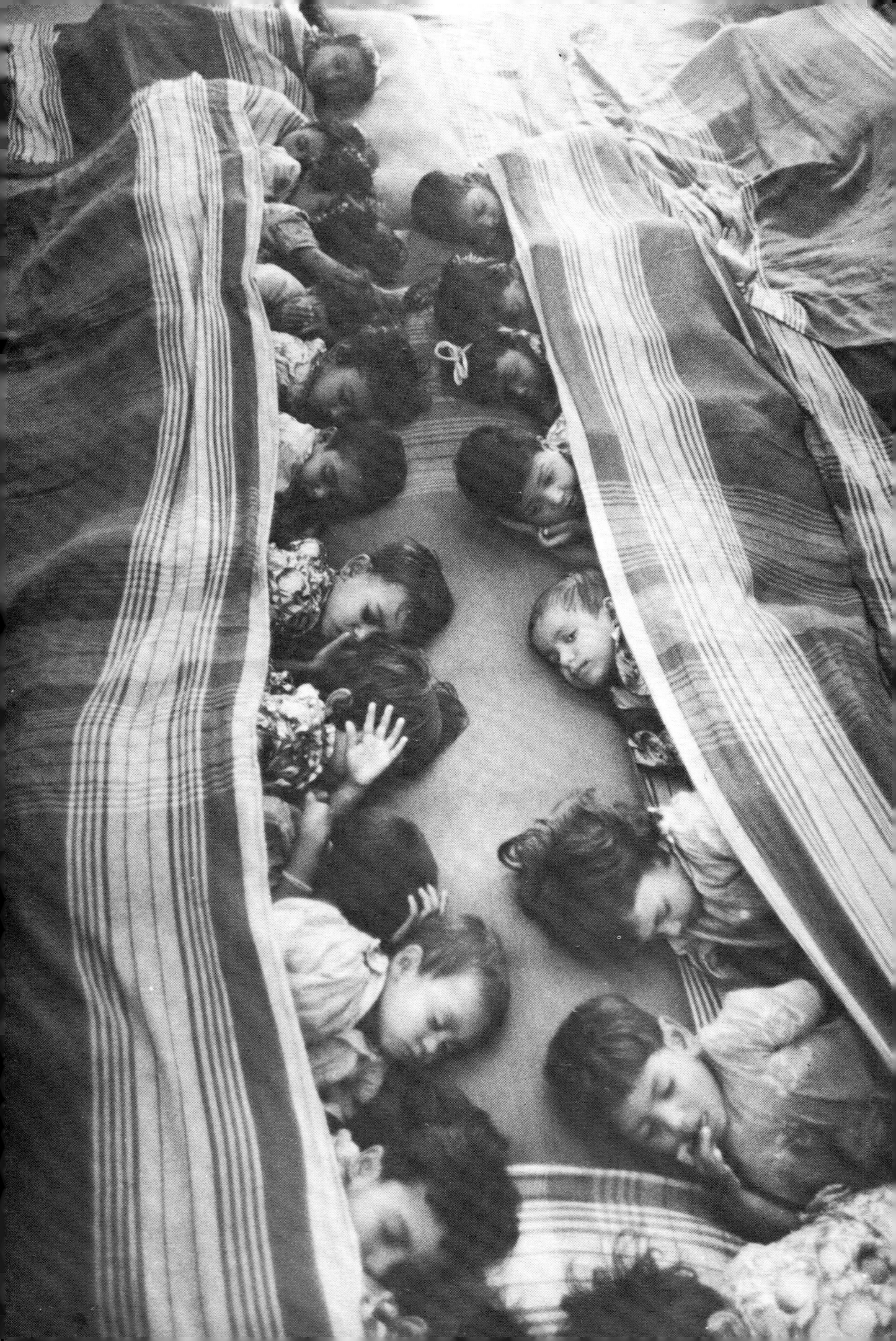

the dangerous symptom of dehydration is easily recognized and can be coped with, even within the family. In Papua, New Guinea, medical auxiliaries have learned to treat dehydration, reducing mortality to the rate of about 1% – which is not worse than average results in many hospitals. In Brazil, there are "rehydration centres," where intravenous injections and perfusions are sometimes prescribed and administered by women who cannot read.

The entire equipment consists of a needle mounted on a tube leading to the infusion set, and a razor blade to shave the scalp when necessary. The result : mortality from dehydration has been reduced to 2%, in spite of poor nutrition and sanitation in isolated villages.

Are doctors always essential ?

Iron deficiency anemia, believed to affect some 700 million people (nearly a fifth of the world's population) is treated by appropriate food or pills containing iron. Where it is particularly widespread, diagnosis is far more costly than systematic treatment of pregnant or lactating women and young children. Once the condition is established, the intervention of medical doctors to treat individual cases is wasteful. Many other examples could be given.

It is true that some diseases are not so readily recognizable and more difficult to treat. But in the total picture of the developing world, they are a minority. A small percentage of respiratory diseases, for instance, is represented by often lethal staphyloccocal pneumonia. Anemia may be difficult to pinpoint with precision. Cancer and heart disease may require complex and costly treatment.

The problem, then, could be put in a different way. When there is no doctor, should the other – the "easy" cases, remain untreated, because it is axiomatic that none but medical doctors should make diagnoses and prescribe treatment ?

Healers who are not biochemists, gynecologists, gastroenterologists, or even medical doctors, can be effective even when they do not understand the precise mechanism of the therapy they prescribe. Come to think of it, how many doctors really understand the mode of action of aspirin ? •

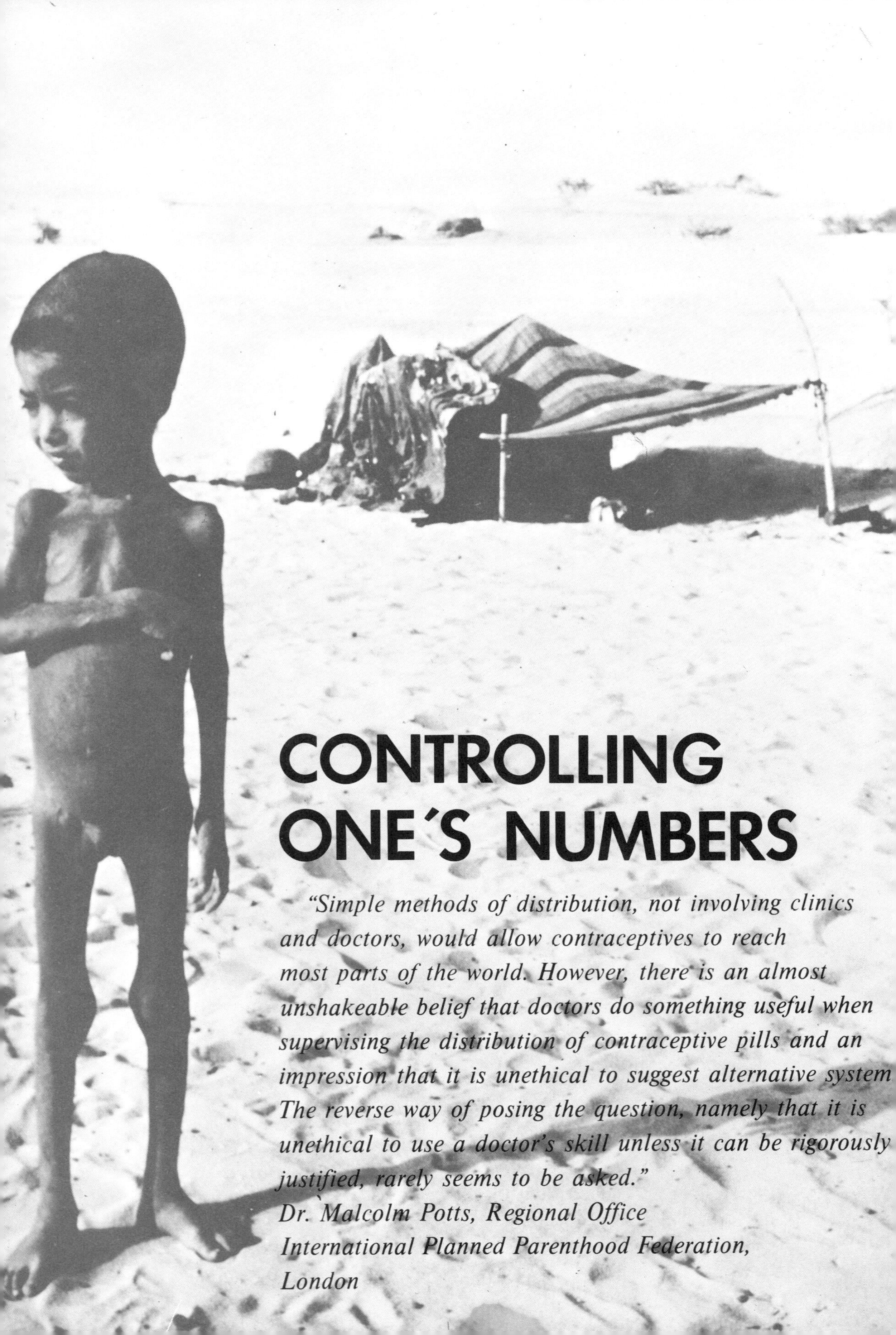

CONTROLLING ONE'S NUMBERS

"Simple methods of distribution, not involving clinics and doctors, would allow contraceptives to reach most parts of the world. However, there is an almost unshakeable belief that doctors do something useful when supervising the distribution of contraceptive pills and an impression that it is unethical to suggest alternative system The reverse way of posing the question, namely that it is unethical to use a doctor's skill unless it can be rigorously justified, rarely seems to be asked."

Dr. Malcolm Potts, Regional Office
International Planned Parenthood Federation,
London

CONTROLLING ONE'S NUMBERS

Man's lifespan and the physiology of his reproductive system indicate a reproductive capacity of about 10 deliveries in a lifetime. Millions of years of evolution have fashioned this system to insure the survival of the species, in circumstances entirely different from those prevailing today.

Not long ago in many parts of the world (and still today in a few parts of the world) the full utilization of this capacity was necessary to insure the survival, to the adult age, of one or two individuals. This is no longer the case. Hygiene, medicine, vaccines, improved living conditions, have made our reproductive system dangerously redundant. Yet, man will retain his reproductive capacities for many thousands of years to come. Evolutionary adaptation is painstakingly slow.

Contraceptives as preventive medicine

It is true that reproduction has to a degree been controlled by custom, but in the past century demographic growth has been so rapid that now only the use of technical means to control one's own reproduction can cope with an increased growth rate that can only be a transitional step in man's history. On the level of a population, contraceptives can be looked upon unemotionally as a means to extend the time taken to conceive.

Contraceptive means are also part of the "right to health" package, because family planning is the only way to control intervals between births with a view of improving the health of the mother and her children, and of insuring the survival of all of the children in a family.

In spite of the emotional context that has surrounded the concept of family planning in recent years, the medical aspects cannot be ignored. Kwashiorkor, the "red child" or "the illness

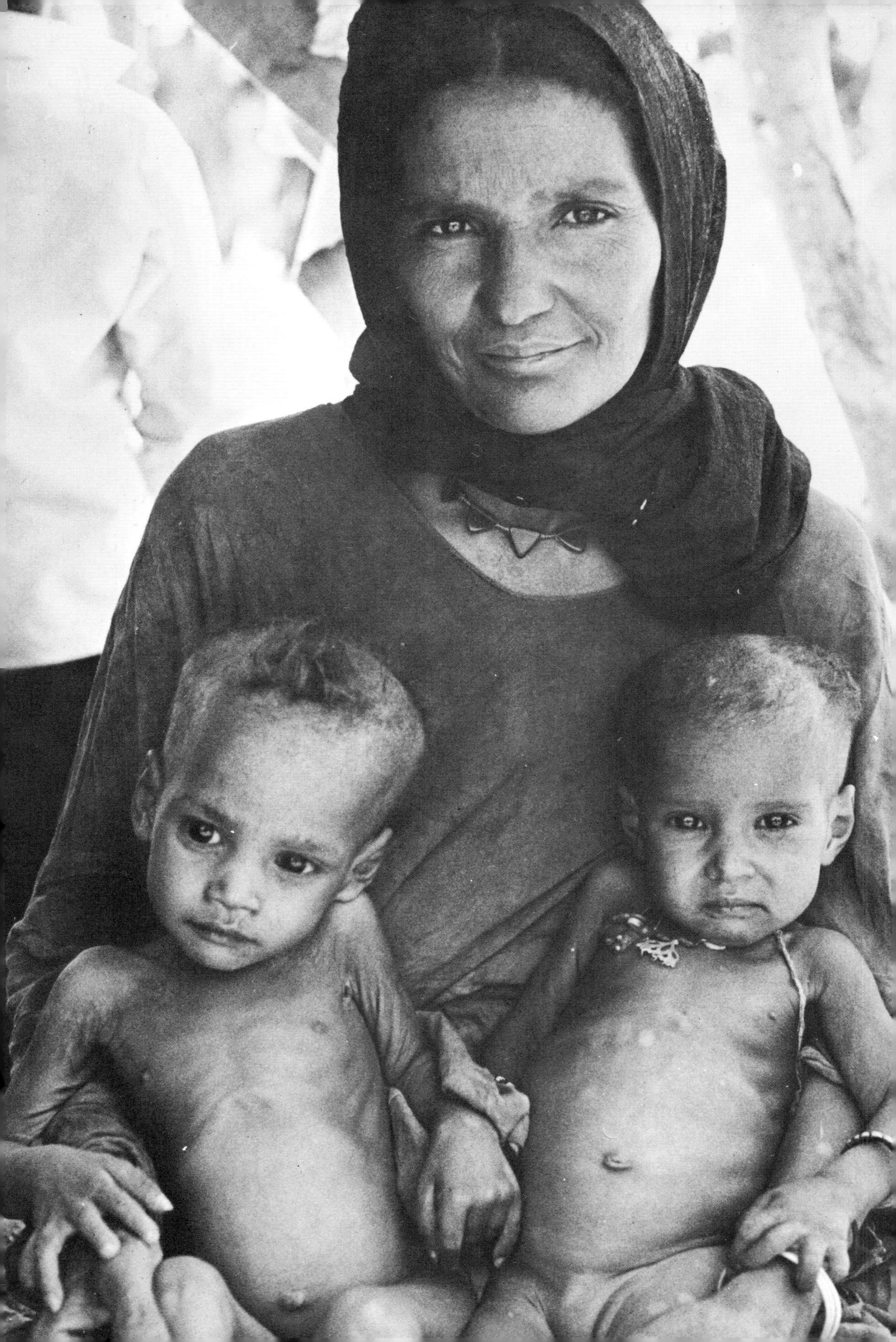

of the deposed baby when the next one is born," is a severe disease caused by protein deficiency usually following abrupt weaning. It is particularly frequent in Africa, but the ill effects of too short intervals between births are known the world over. It has been shown that in the United States, just as in poorer countries, there is a considerable decrease in infant malnutrition when the interval between births exceeds two or three years. The rate of infant mortality is four times less when a second pregnancy occurs two years after the first birth, than when it takes place only four months after it. Family planning, in other words, is effective prevention against kwashiorkor.

A choice, not a limitation

Thus family planning need not be identified with limitation of family size or Malthusian politics, and this particularly true in under-populated developing countries. It can mean, on the contrary, increased family size – increased, at least, with respect to the number of survivors. It is part of health care.

Modern contraceptive methods are the outcome of biological and medical research, and it is not surprising that medical doctors have tended to monopolize not only the technical, but the moral aspects of family planning. They have often opposed simple and

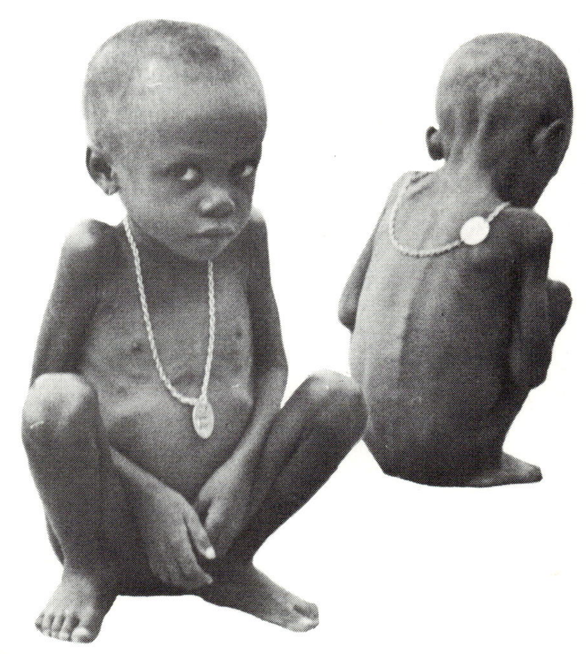

Not only drought, but a rapid population increase, have contributed to famine in the Sahelian zone of Africa. It is known that child mortality increases when pregnancies occur in rapid succession.

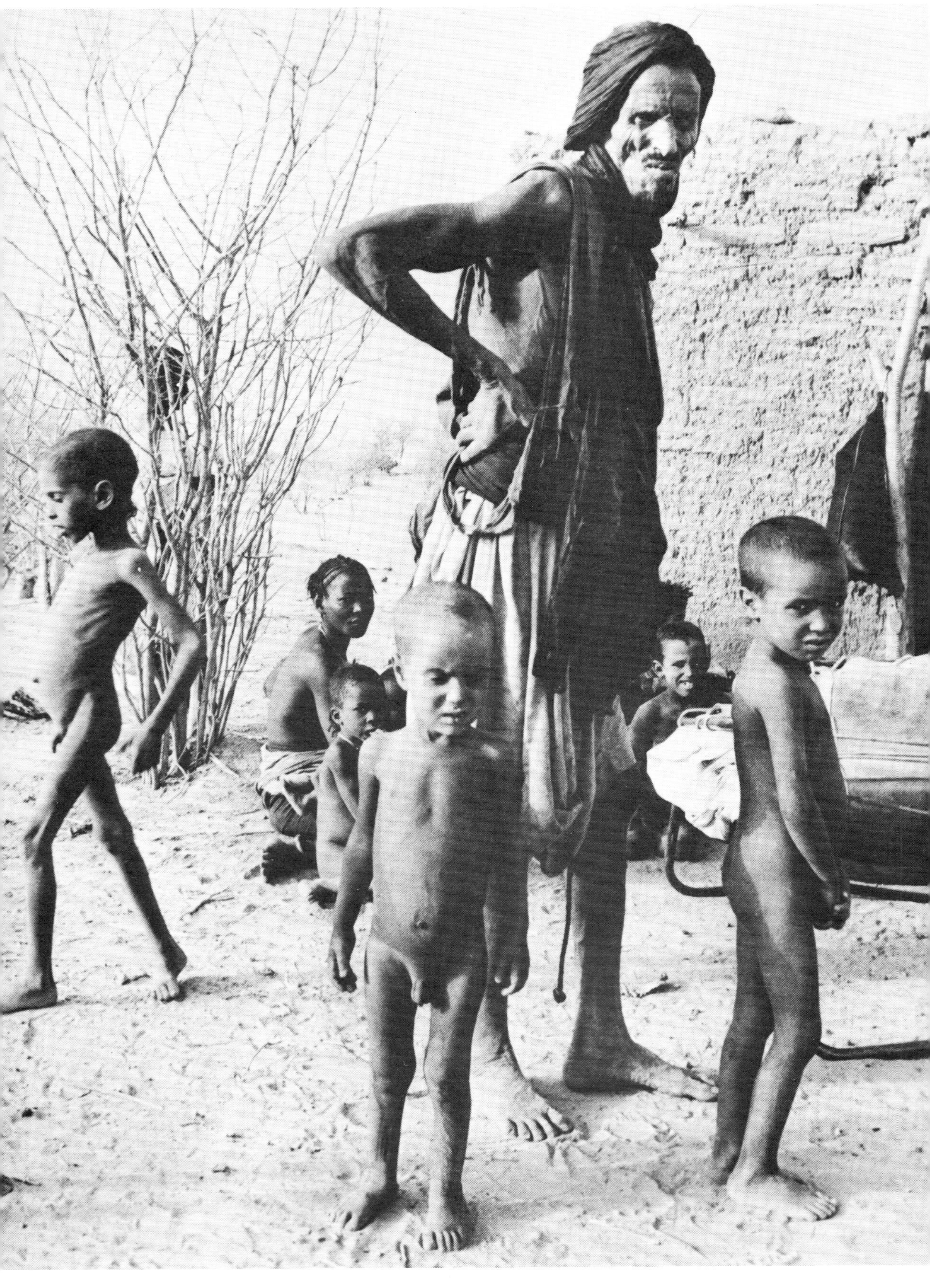

straightforward distribution of contraceptives and of information about their use. Yet, the use of a pill or a condom does not really require the supervision or assistance of a graduate of a medical faculty.

Simple techniques, even for abortion

The introduction of a medical doctor into the family planning programs of rural areas can become a drawback, particularly when the doctor is a stranger and does not remain in the area, while a village health worker, a mayor, or any other trusted member of the group, is familiar with his people, their problems, their attitudes, their taboos. It is easy for him to learn the do's and don'ts of family planning methods. Trials in several countries (Indonesia, Korea, Pakistan, Barbados, Guatemala and others) have shown that auxiliary personnel can not only distribute condoms and deliver pills, but learn to perform pelvic examinations and insert intra-uterine devices. The example of China shows that even abortions, performed with simple techniques, do not require the skills of a highly trained medical practitioner ●

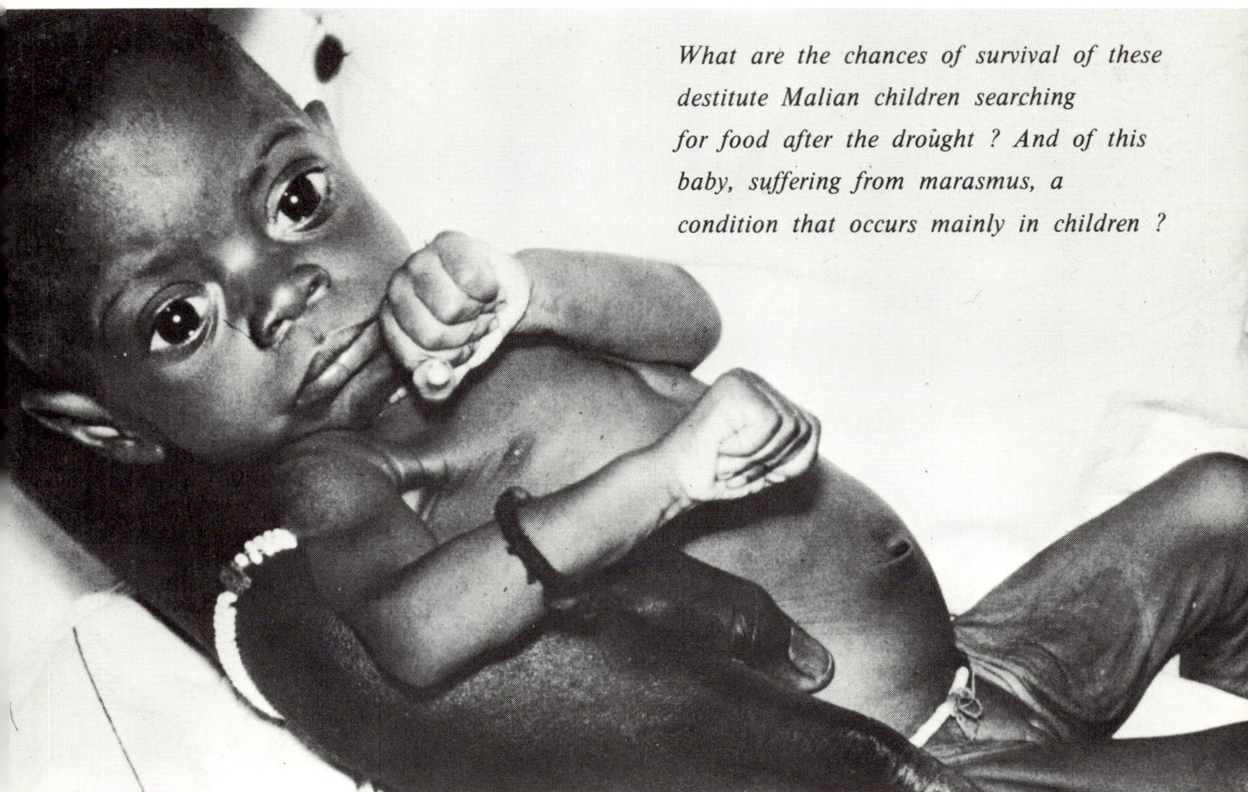

What are the chances of survival of these destitute Malian children searching for food after the drought ? And of this baby, suffering from marasmus, a condition that occurs mainly in children ?

THE STORY OF A MONOPOLY

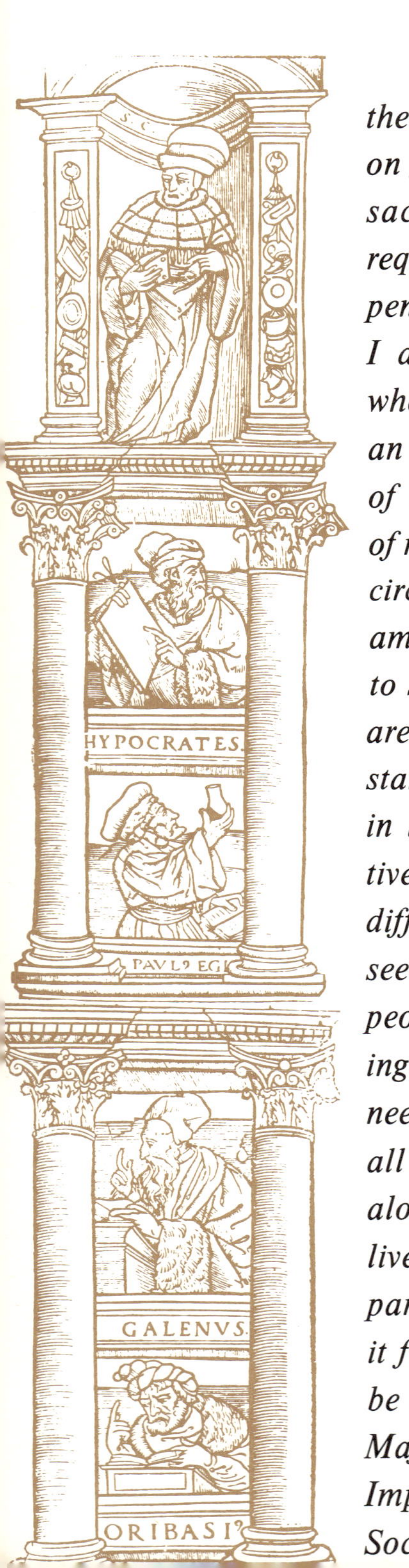

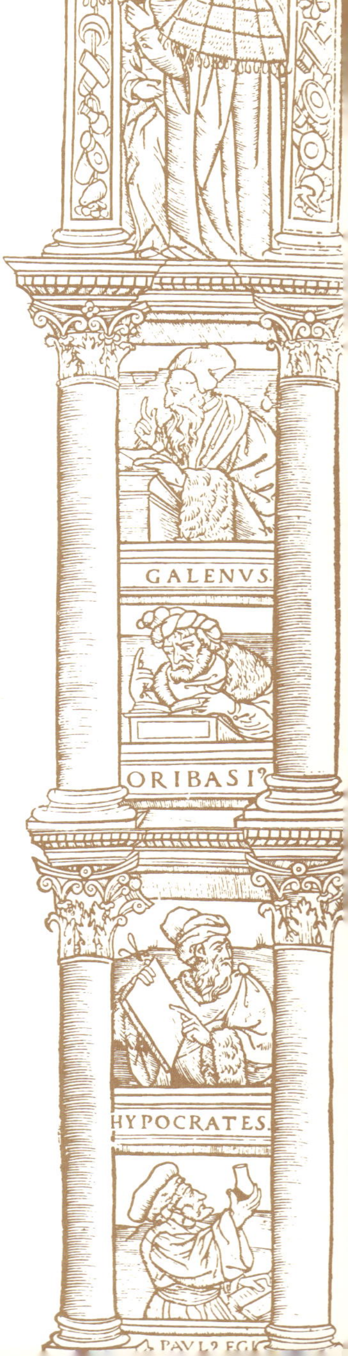

The facts of the situation provide the best answer to those who argue on grounds of high principle that the sacred character of human life requires that medical care be dispensed by doctors alone. Where, may I ask, are these moralizing doctors when village children fall ill or suffer an injury ? If they promote this kind of ethics in big cities, in the schools of medicine and in other distinguished circles, while millions, especially among children, continue to die and to suffer in areas where none of them are prepared to go ? One can understand that a doctor finds difficulty in living in remote areas under relatively primitive conditions. But it is difficult to accept that they should seek to prevent others, mainly the people most concerned, from bringing health services to the areas in need... If human life is sacred, as we all believe it to be, and if doctors alone are entitled to deal with human lives, and if finally they are not prepared to assume that responsibility, it follows that something else should be done.

Majid Rahnema, special advisor, Imperial Organization for Social Services, Iran

THE STORY OF A MONOPOLY

Medicine is the oldest, largest, most widespread, wealthiest, and perhaps the most powerful single monopoly in the world today.

Such a statement need not be taken as a criticism or a condemnation. It corresponds to the classical definition of a monopoly as the exclusive control of the supply of any commodity or service in a given market. The commodity is health care ; the market, the world.

From 1224 to date

Western medicine can be said to have existed since the beginning of the 13th century, when the Medical School of Salerno was organized, at a time when Arabic medicine, still dominant, was on the decline. The monopoly itself could be dated more precisely to the year 1224, when Emperor Frederick II of the Holy Roman Empire decreed that no one should pratice medicine without having passed an examination before the masters of the Medical School of Salerno. This monopoly has been maintained for seven and a half centuries.

Today, accepted medical practitioners are, as a rule, graduates of Western-style medical faculties that have, all over the world, very similar requirements and approximately equivalent degrees. Practitioners who are not approved by the medical schools are usually considered to be quacks, and sometimes are meted out punishment not too dissimilar to that decreed in the 13th century of "imprisonment and confiscation of goods."

This monopoly has not developed as a result of collusion, nor from the desire for power or wealth. In the beginning it seems just to have happened ; the reasons for its survival and growth are debatable. It has set standards that have been, at any given time,

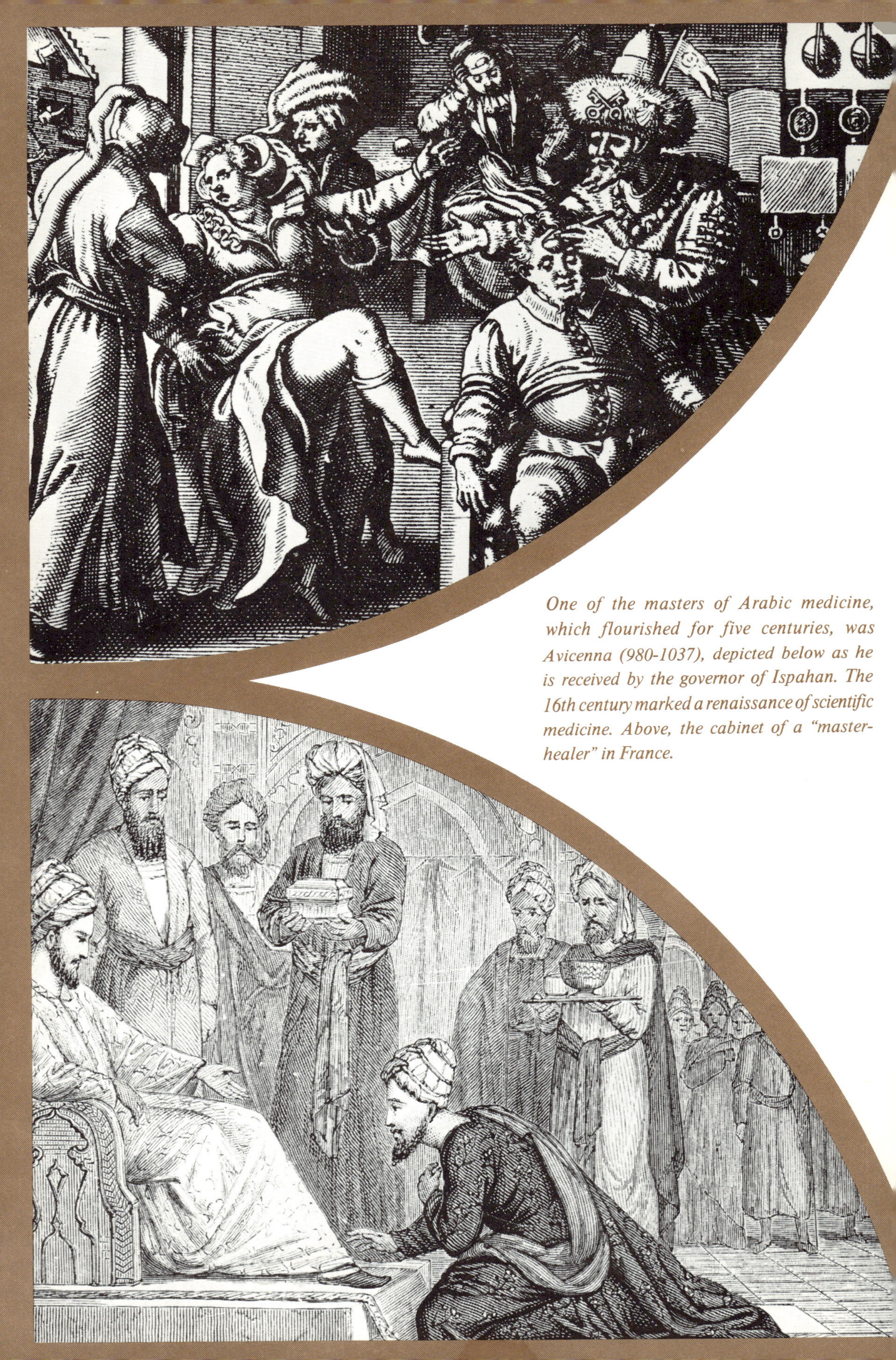

One of the masters of Arabic medicine, which flourished for five centuries, was Avicenna (980-1037), depicted below as he is received by the governor of Ispahan. The 16th century marked a renaissance of scientific medicine. Above, the cabinet of a "master-healer" in France.

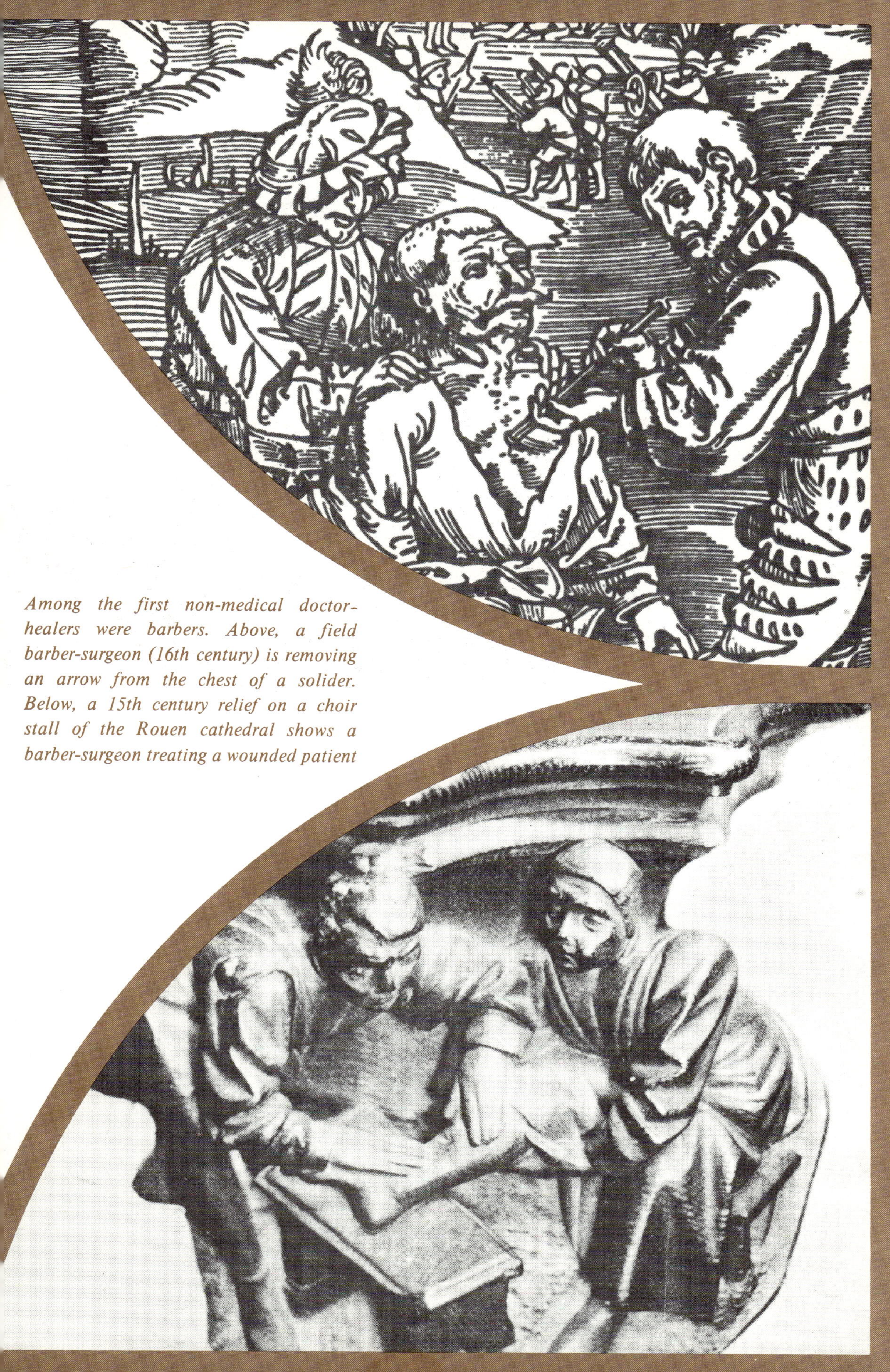

Among the first non-medical doctor-healers were barbers. Above, a field barber-surgeon (16th century) is removing an arrow from the chest of a solider. Below, a 15th century relief on a choir stall of the Rouen cathedral shows a barber-surgeon treating a wounded patient

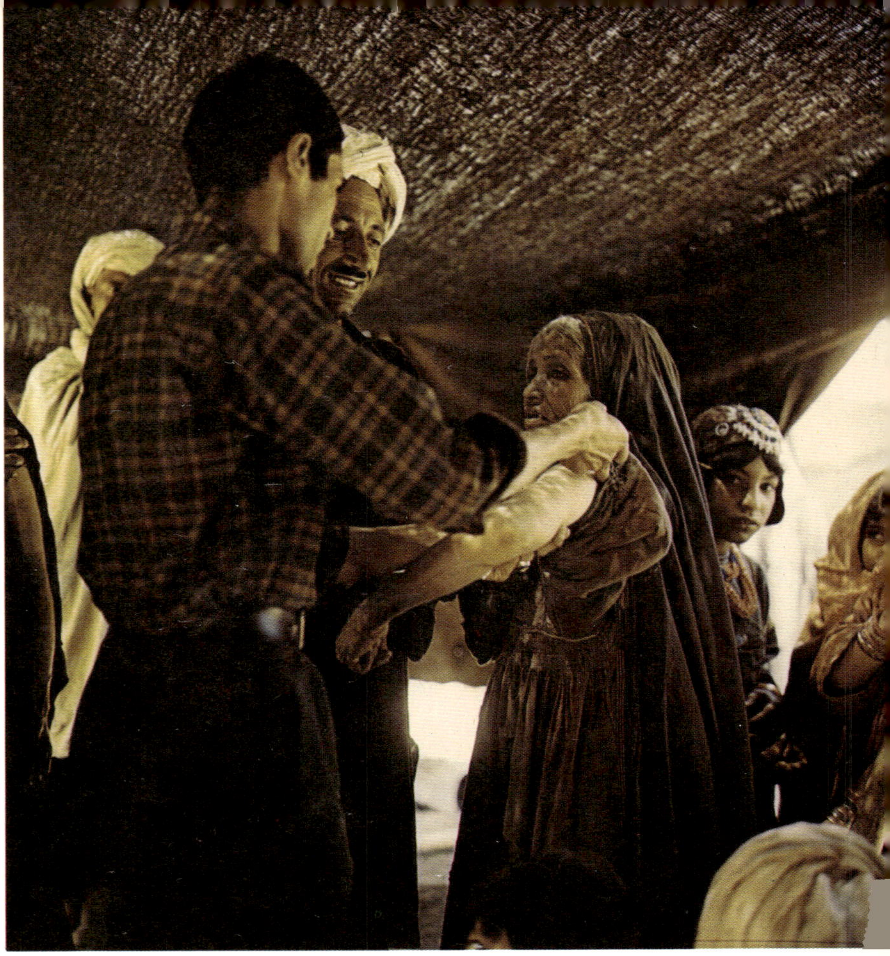

*A health worker carries on a
vaccination campaign in
Afghanistan.*

*Medicine among American Indians,
as seen by a Frenchman
in the 18th century.*

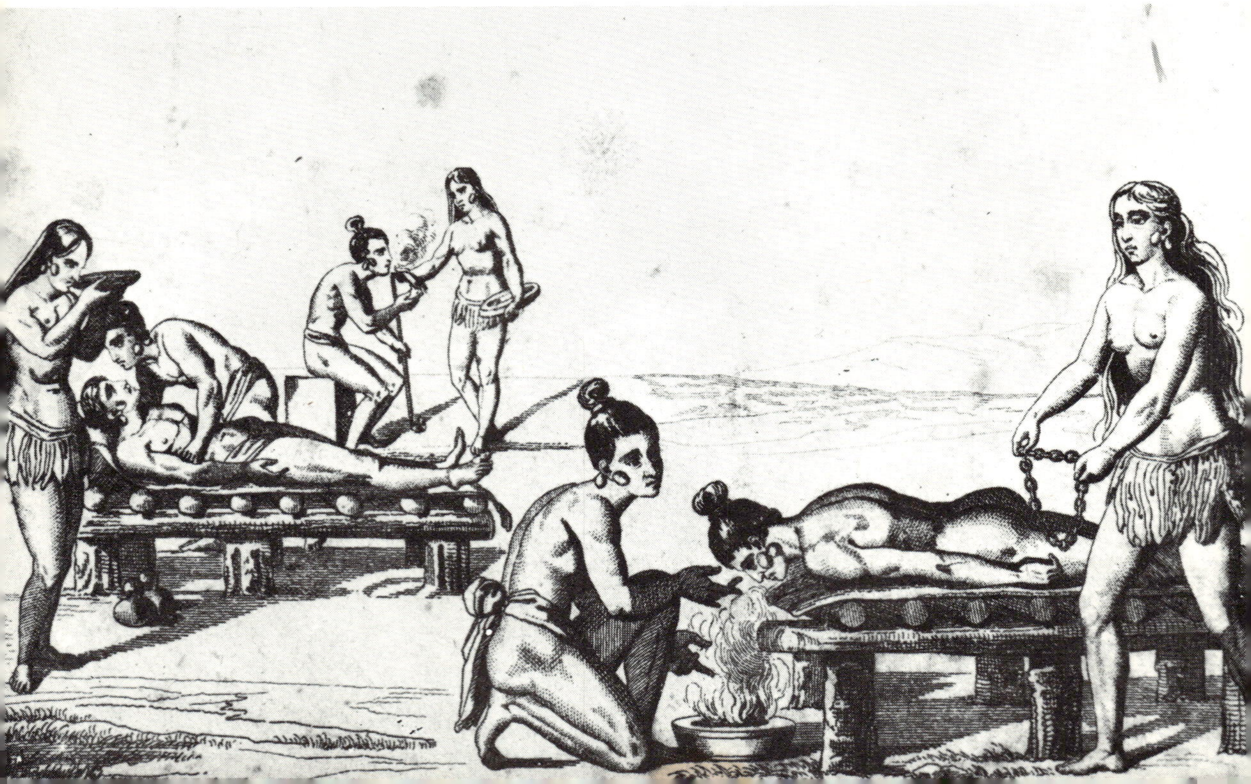

the best available, and it has had a powerful, beneficial effect in restricting charlatans.

Membership in the medical establishment gives the right to diagnose diseases and treat patients and, depending upon the social and political setting where medicine is practiced, to be paid a salary or to collect a fee for services rendered. In many cases the fee is set by the profession itself or by the individual practitioner ; in others it is predetermined ; the fee is paid either by individuals, or by society. None of these differences really detract from the monopolistic situation.

A sudden discontinuity

Membership does not give all members equal right, status, or income, and this is understandable. A heart surgeon may place a valve, a neurosurgeon extract a brain tumor, while a general practitioner does neither. Thus within the profession, there are levels of expertise, and limitations, often corresponding to levels of status and of income.

What may seem surprising is that levels of expertise do not continue below a certain point. There is a discontinuity. A general practitioner can treat ulcers, but no one who has not graduated from medical school should − in principle − diagnose a head cold and prescribe an aspirin.

Pharmacists are a tolerated exception, but there is a subtle yet important difference, in that pharmacists are not paid for the disgnostic service, but earn their living from profits on the drugs they sell and may occasionally prescribe.

There are, of course, other exceptions. One is self-medication, widely tolerated and even encouraged for certain categories of diseases and certain drugs. These drugs are sometimes openly advertised, and the diagnostic steps as well as the therapeutic dosages are described to the public in newspaper and television advertisements. As a consequence lay people, by advising others, or telling them of their own experience with such or such medicine, often diagnose diseases and prescribe treatment, and this, too, is tolerated, as long as the lay person does not ask for a fee for the service performed. The medical profession cannot tolerate that an "unqualified" healer be paid, and here again it reveals its monopolistic position.

There is yet another exception, that of the non-medical doctor who is a professional healer. This term may appear to be contradictory, because professionalism in the field of health care almost automatically attributed to medical doctors. The term *"professional"* is used here in its reference to an occupation providing livelihood, as opposed to amateurism. The professional non-doctor healer has existed for a long time, and for a long time he has been repressed by the medical profession. Today, his numbers are increasing, and it is likely that before long, the number of non-medical doctor-healers will exceed that of medical doctors.

Such healers are known by a variety of names, and their functions and responsibilities vary from country to country and region to region. They are medical assistants or auxiliaries, health officers or promoters, feldshers or barefoot doctors, medex or health extension workers, African doctors or health provosts.

In the 16th century and even before, feldshers (from the German for field barbers) received additional training to act as military medical men. They shaved their masters, but also followed them in battle and wielded the scalpel – an instrument not unlike the barber's knife. Peter the Great officially turned field barbers into part-time health workers to compensate for the shortage of trained physicians in the Russian armies. Feldshers in the Soviet Union today have retained this role, and have been integrated into the health care delivery system. After the Soviet revolution, many were upgraded to physicians, but new feldsher schools were created. Today they may act as doctors' assistants, laboratory technicians, public health specialists, occupational health specialists but, in smaller towns and rural areas, they substitute for medical doctors and, in their absence, act on their own authority.

In Jamaica, since the 17th century, physicians' assistants who had served apprenticeship and passed examinations could sell herbal preparations and drugs, and became independent medical healers in rural areas. After emancipation in the 19th century, formal training for dispensers was set up, until a "proper" medical school was established in 1954.

The Jamaican pattern, with variations, was repeated in many African countries during colonial times. An outstanding case in point is that of Senegal, where the *Ecole Africaine de Médecine* was founded by the French in 1918, and produced, by 1951, more than 800 *médecins africains,* each having followed four years of training in simple obstetrical and surgical procedures, preventive medicine, public health and sanitation.

Most of them worked "in the bush," where European doctors were seldom seen. They were effective not only because they cared for their own people in conditions these people had been accustomed to, but perhaps also because they were not allowed to set up private practice in town, nor accepted as medical practitioners abroad. Similar systems were adopted in Madagascar, Nigeria, Zanzibar (now part of Tanzania) and Fiji.

Medicine as a status symbol

Another example is that of India, which had, by 1948, 14 medical colleges on the university level, and more than 20 medical schools that offered four years of training to high school graduates who became "licensed medical practioners" or "sub-assistant surgeons." They could practice medicine on their own, and were commonly referred to as "doctors."

When colonies achieved independence many of these systems crumbled away. Local governments felt in many cases that the "auxiliary doctor" system had been set up so that "proper" doctoring would be reserved for Europeans. Once independent, the European-trained indigenous medical doctors understandably tended to perpetuate the colonial medical monopoly (to which they belonged) either by rejecting non-doctor healers, or by upgrading them to their level, without realizing that they might be suppressing something that corresponded to the needs of the people far better than a totally imported system. It is undeniable also that medical degrees became status symbols, like tall buildings, steel mills, and limousines.

Thus the *Ecole Africaine de Médecine* has ceased to exist, to be replaced by the "proper" medical faculty of Dakar ; some of the *médecins africains* have been upgraded, while the others are gradually disappearing. In India, all of the medical schools have been transformed into colleges, and new colleges have been added, so that India today is one of the world's major exporters of medical doctors to rich countries. Many large population groups have remained without any medical care at all. Native healers that existed in almost every country have to a great extent been prevented from practicing in the open. Yet, some of these, too, could have learned enough modern medical technology to become "medical healers" and be integrated into a health system. As Anthropologist Margaret Mead has pointed out in a study carried out for UNESCO : "The introduction of medicine has meant a loss of faith in the known, and when the new medicine proved too expensive, people found themselves without any medicine."

Monopolizing the simplest tools

The most ironically tragic aspect of the failure to provide adequate medical coverage in many countries is that medical technology in the past few decades has become such that most of the major diseases in developing areas are easily recognized, and the means of treating or preventing them are known. There is no need for a post-graduate specialist to diagnose the pattern of diseases that carry the heaviest toll. Ivan Illich, director of the Intercultural Documentation Centre in Cuernavaca, Mexico, has aptly decribed the situation in a few words : "The paradox is that the more the tool becomes simple, the more the medical profession persists in monopolizing it. The more the initiation of the therapist is lengthy, the more people become dependent upon him for rendering the most elementary care."

Unfortunately, it must be added that in many developing countries, the hope for the population to receive adequate health care is also thwarted by the attitudes of the elite, devoted to Western medical standards. This has two consequences – the first being that these standards become incorporated into the national goal. Medical schools are designed in terms of prestige symbols, rather than to improve the health of the people. This may represent an enormous drain on the limited resources allocated to the health of the population.

A second consequence is a form of collusion of the elite with the medical monopoly, once more to the detriment of the people. An example is provided by the close examination of the health budget of one African country (and there are, probably, others where a similar situation prevails). In that country, nearly half of the health budget is spent to give Western-style treatment to an elite representing at most a few percent of the total population. A widespread practice (sometimes encouraged by "donor" countries, as a way of maintaining a friendly relationship with the decision-making elite) is known under the euphemism of "sanitary evacuation." This means that a civil servant, usually of a high level, is flown to Europe for the treatment of a more or less real disease, and put up in a costly clinic. Sometimes part of the family comes along to stay in a nearby hotel. The expense, of course, is absorbed by the health budget of the African country, but that isn't all. Some time later, the grateful African official invites the treating doctor on a "study trip" to his sunny country. The trip may start with a brief visit to a hospital, but usually includes a lengthier "relaxation time" in the form of a safari in a national park or a stay at a seaside resort. The cost is also listed under the country's health expenditures ; the medical monopoly is reinforced, and the health care gap widens ●

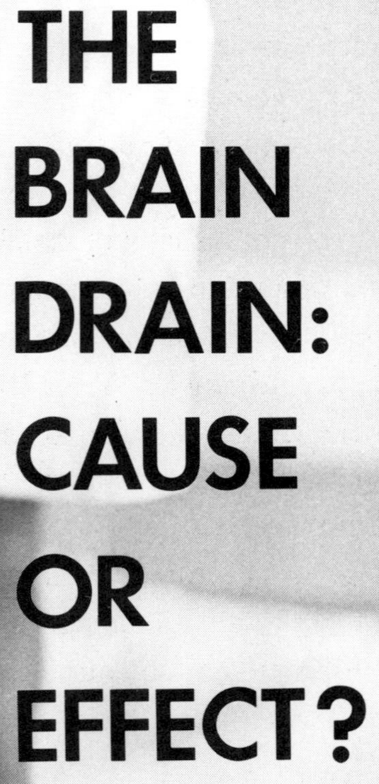

THE BRAIN DRAIN: CAUSE OR EFFECT?

"Of the 16 689 physicians newly licensed (in the
United States in 1973), 7 419, or almost one half, were
graduates of foreign medical schools, reflecting
for the seventh consecutive year a substantial increase
in the number of foreign physicians taking state board
examinations."
Press release,
American Medical Association

THE BRAIN DRAIN:
CAUSE OR EFFECT ?

A Nigerian medical doctor, graduate of the faculty of Ibadan, is quite understandably tempted when he receives a fellowship to specialize in paediatrics in London or Edinburgh. He may leave with the intention of returning to his country, but having completed the post-graduate specialty, he will undoubtedly realize that the conditions to practice it as he has learned it are better in Europe than in his own country. He is, just as understandably, tempted to accept a staff position in a British hospital. Eventually, he may acquire British nationality.

A British graduate, in turn, may well be interested in post-graduate work in Harvard or New York. Should he select a specialty not favored by American physicians (proctology, for instance) he will have no difficulty in obtaining a staff position and settling in North America, where his income will be considerably higher than it would be under the National Health Service scheme in England.

It may be that a few American doctors, sponsored by a government agency or a private foundation, may follow a course in tropical medicine and travel to Africa to practice in isolated regions, or to teach in an African medical school. But, with very few exceptions, these doctors will return home rather than settle in primitive conditions that are foreign to their way of life, and where the cultural and language gaps as well as the lack of facilities make it impossible to practice the kind of medicine they have been taught.

This circuitous path of medical doctors around the globe may take different forms, but it always runs in the same general direction, from the less affluent to the more affluent countries. Thus in 1972, 447 British physicians took the test of the U.S. Educational Council for Foreign Medical Graduates (ECFMG) and 420 of these passed the one-day examination to obtain the certification required to enter the intern and residency programs approved by the American

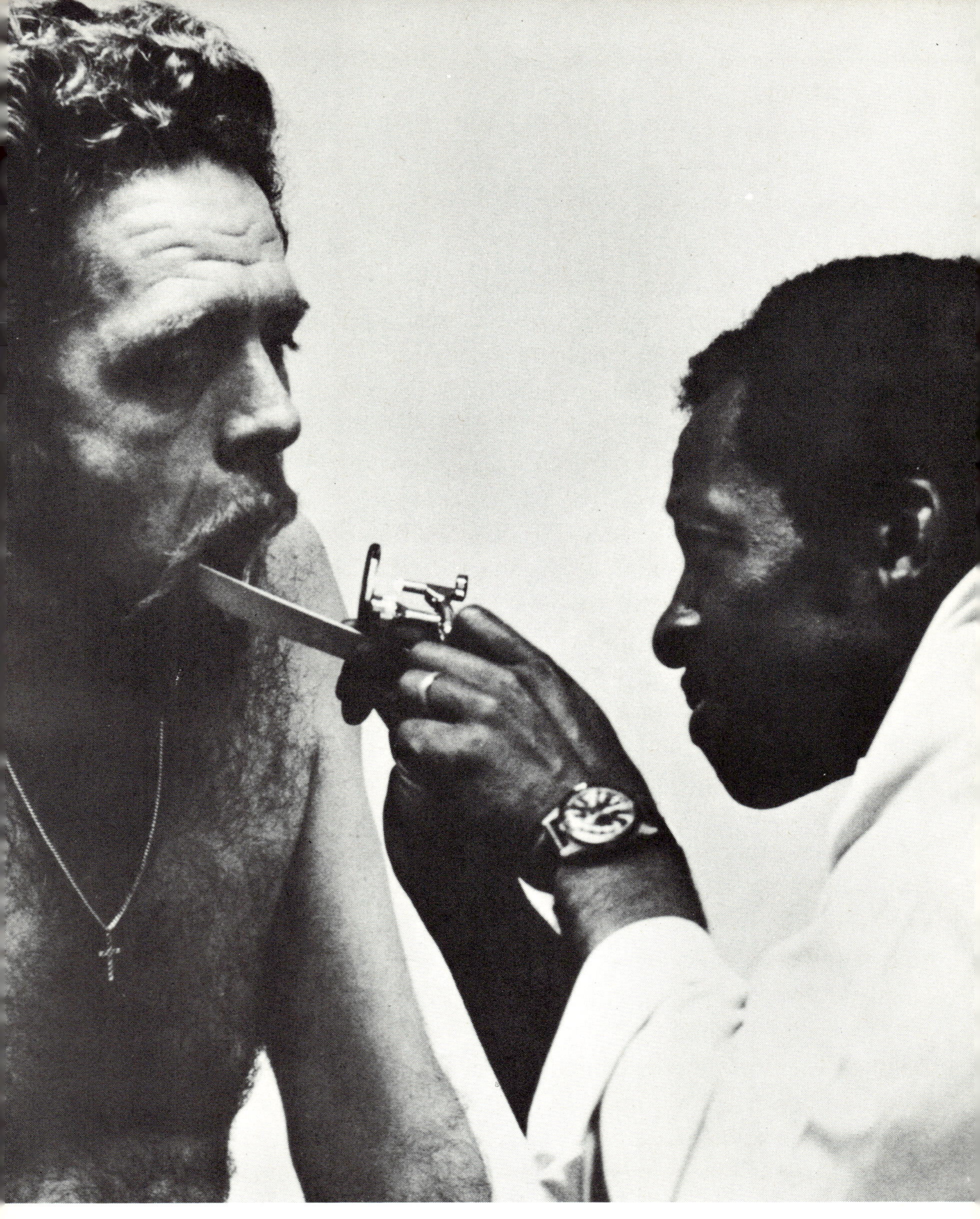

Rich countries are major importers of
medical doctors from poor ones. In
the U.S. and Canada, about one
fifth of the licensed physicians
are foreign medical graduates.

Medical Association. During the same year, 201 Nigerians took the ECFMG test, and 110 passed it.

Viewed from the American perspective, this number may seem small in comparison to some 330 000 licensed physicians in the country. But it adds up – still by the end of 1972 – to a total of 68 000 graduates of foreign medical schools (representing about one fifth of the nation's physicians) licensed to practice in the United States. There were another 11 000 in Canada.

Viewed from the other side, that of developing countries, this represents a huge drain. Nigeria has less than 3 000 physicians, with a ratio estimated at one per 20 000 people. Since most of these physicians practice in larger cities, the ratio for the majority of the population is between one to 50 000 and one to 100 000, which means that 100 Nigerian physicians who leave for the United States or elsewhere could provide at least some medical coverage to a population between one half and one million.

Far from slowing down, this drain away from the poor countries has been increasing. In 1947, 43.7 % of the physicians emigrating to the United States came from Europe. A year ago, this percentage was down to 12 - while   Asia contributed two thirds of all foreign medical graduates coming to the U.S.

Countries like the Philippines and Iran lose to the United States and other industrial countries about one third of their crop of medical graduates. In 1972, more than 4 000 Indian physicians applied for the ECFMG, and 1 667 passed it. The respective figures were 481 and 207 for Brazil ; 1 150 and 481 for Taiwan ; 121 and 42 for Guatemala ; 131 and 45 for El Salvador ; 149 and 45 for Bangladesh ; 430 and 121 for Colombia ; and 972 and 245 for Pakistan. It has been estimated that 8 to 10 medical faculties in India, and two in Central America, function exclusively to supply doctors to the United States and other rich countries.

Mr. Majid Rahnema, former Minister of Science and Higher Education in Iran, and now special advisor to the Imperial Organization for Social Services, writes that "the 1971 figures provided by Pahlavi University show that while Iranian universities produced 600 doctors that year, 675 doctors left Iran for abroad. I hope and believe that was an exceptional year, but there is no denying the seriousness of the problem."

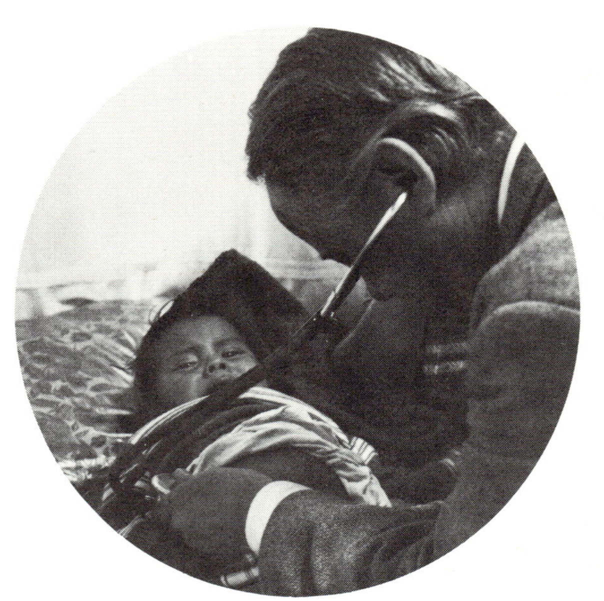

American and European medical doctors sometimes practice in developing countries. But how long will they stay before returning home ?

A medical assistant, like Haile Aenege of Ethiopia (below) directs a health center in his country -- and is not likely to emigrate to set up practice elsewhere.

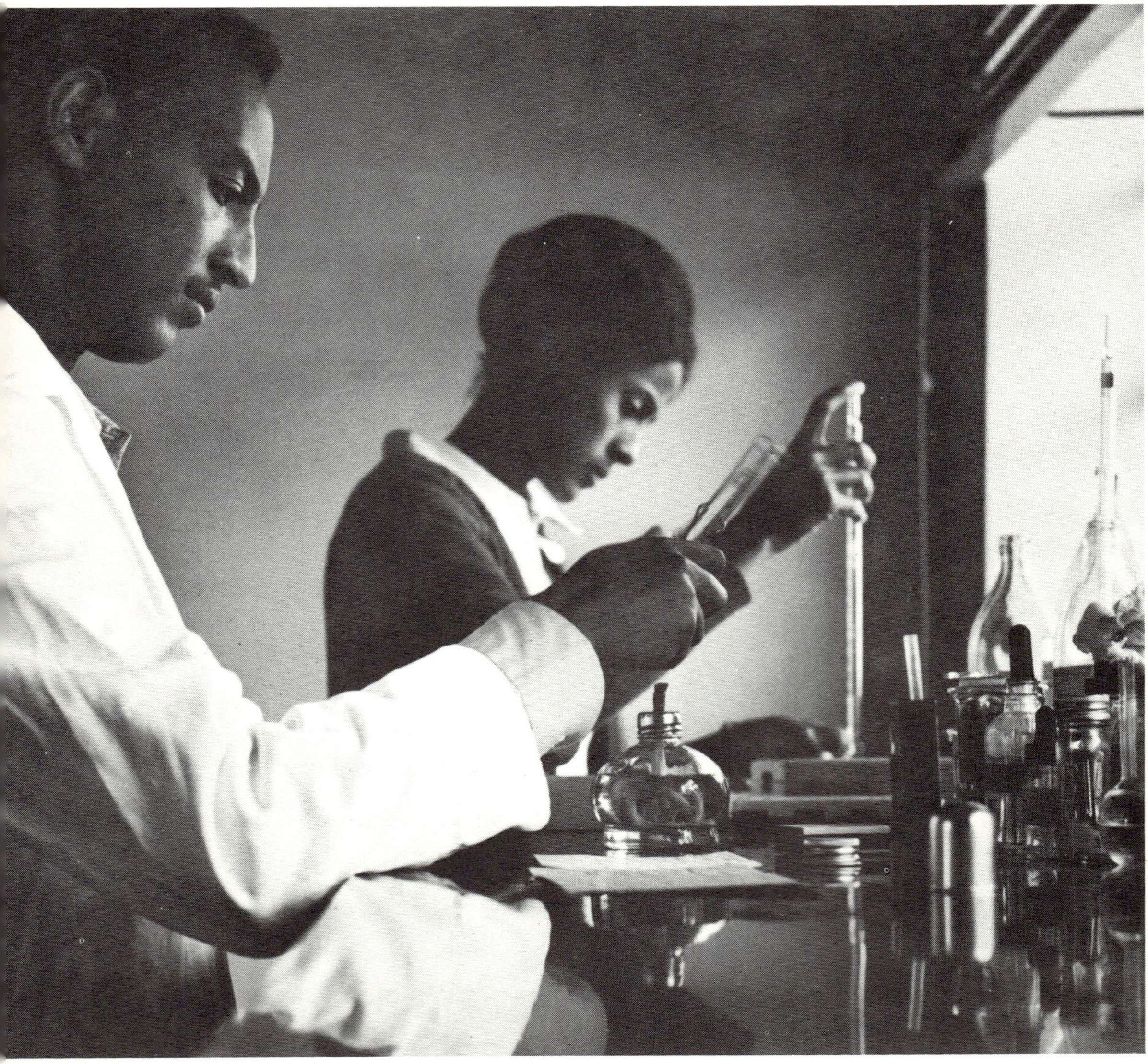

Dr. Alex Gerber, of the University of Southern California Medical School, estimates that the input of foreign medical graduates represents, for the United States alone, $430 million a year in reverse foreign aid, much of it from countries that can little afford it. This annual input comes in addition to a capital investment of about four billion dollars which the United States has saved by not having to set up the medical schools and affiliated university hospitals required to produce more than 4000 medical doctors a year. "The continuing brain drain of physicians from underdeveloped countries to our shores," he writes, "leaves no doubt about who is helping whom medically and this blatant foreign aid in reverse policy is rapidly becoming a national disgrace."

Another form of "cost accounting," by the Department of Community Health of Pahlavi University shows that future earnings of an Iranian physician who emigrates to the United States amount to an average of $573,000 – that is, $91.7 million for the 160 who were licensed in 1970 alone. This is what they are "worth" to the U.S. – and what they do not contribute to their own country. Extrapolating this to some 80 000 foreign MDs who have settled in North America in the past 20 years, this amounts to a staggering "reverse foreign aid" bill of $45 billion !

This exercise in accounting gives an idea of the magnitude of the problem. But is the brain drain really a drain ? Dr. Henry Mason, of the AMA's Division of Medical Education, concludes that it is, in fact, not a drain but an overflow of physicians who can find no proper place for their talents at home. Young graduates, understandably, want the best possible career. They are trained to practice what could be termed "luxury medicine," and they go where there is a demand for it. Advanced countries hesitate to close their doors, and developing ones, to imprison the MDs they have produced at such a high cost.

It seems amazing that poor countries continue to produce healers for rich countries. And, while negotiating new prices for some of their natural resources, go on exporting for free a resource they are, themselves, so much in need of. But such is the prestige value of a Western medical faculty, and the power of the monopoly, that this is likely to continue for many years to come ●

THE DOCTOR - HEALER RELATIONSHIP

"Physicians are like kings,
They brook no contradiction."
John Webster
English dramatist

THE DOCTOR-HEALER RELATIONSHIP

There are few statistics on diagnostic errors by medical practitioners. There are even fewer, however, attempting to compare diagnosis and treatment by medical doctors on one hand, and non-doctor on the other. The very thought of such a comparison seems to be almost irreverent and somehow unethical. One comparative study, carried out by Dr. Hossain A. Ronaghy, of the Department of Community Medicine of Pahlavi University, Shiraz, Iran, gives rather surprising results. In the study, 244 consecutive patients were seen independently both by a physician and by an "auxiliary" with no medical training (he was a young economist who had worked as a clinic coordinator for a year).

Each patient was first seen by the auxiliary, who recorded his impressions of the patient's problems and his suggestions for treatment. The patient was then interviewed and treated by a physician, who had not been informed of the auxiliary's "diagnosis." The results were then compared.

It turned out that only in four cases did the auxiliary miss a potentially serious problem, and none of these was a life-and-death matter. Most doctors will agree that even for a medical practitioner, a margin of error of less than 2% cannot be considered as excessive.

The comparison is unexpectedly favourable to the unlicensed non-doctor, and Dr. Ronaghy recognizes that the number of cases examined is not sufficient for the study to be "statistically significant."

A similar study was carried out in Guatemala by a graduate student of the Department of Community Medicine of the University of Kentucky College of Medicine. He found that "healers" with a few weeks' training make the proper diagnosis and prescribe appropriate treatment in about 70% of the cases. The investigator found that sometimes the treatment prescribed by the healer was incomplete, and that sometimes unnecessary extras were added, but he also concluded that no patient was harmed by a wrong treatment.

Few doctors who have worked with auxiliaries, or have seen them work, find them useless or harmful. Prof. Pierre Pène, director of the Tropical Medicine and Health Research and Teaching Unit at the University of Aix-Marseille, who has long practiced and taught in Africa, finds that the vanishing *médecins africains* have been immensely useful to their country. In a study of 15 African states, he has found that medical density in rural areas is between one physician for 30 000 people and one for 100 000. He concludes : "In spite of the efforts deployed by goverments, rural areas are, and shall long remain, under-medicated. It is for these rural areas that should be formulated, and solved in a realistic manner, the problem of the formation and utilization of an auxiliary medical personnel."

Yet, little has been done on national levels. Why ? According to the World Health Organization's "Organization study on methods of promoting the development of basic health services" (1973) :

"A pattern is emerging of less or least utilization of health services in areas that have the least sufficient services. There is a shortage of trained staff at all levels ; but countries that have insufficient staff show the greatest maldistribution within the country, and appear to have the highest emigration rate... There have been few large-scale attempts to find, introduce and supervise a health service staffed mainly by health auxiliaries responsible for primary care. For example, the barefoot doctor idea is an interesting one deserving greater attention. If the peripheral services have clearly stated technical functions consistent with the national goals, proper supervision, and a referral system related to the more specialized health service resources and the needs and demands of the community, it would appear probable that coverage and utilization would be improved and a greater return would result from their use. It could be said that the way in which such a service could be run is already known and that what is lacking is a national will and a manner of overcoming the entrenched opposition of organized medicine" ●

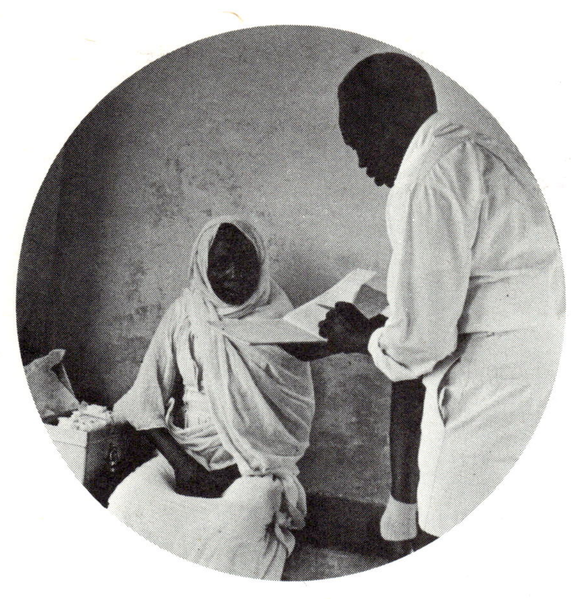

In most of the countries where medical auxiliary programs have been initiated, good results have been obtained. Left : in Sudan, an auxiliary discusses the birth of a child with a midwife. Below : in Algeria, the Institute of Health Technology.

Bottom : In India, instructions about family planning are given by a trained health worker.

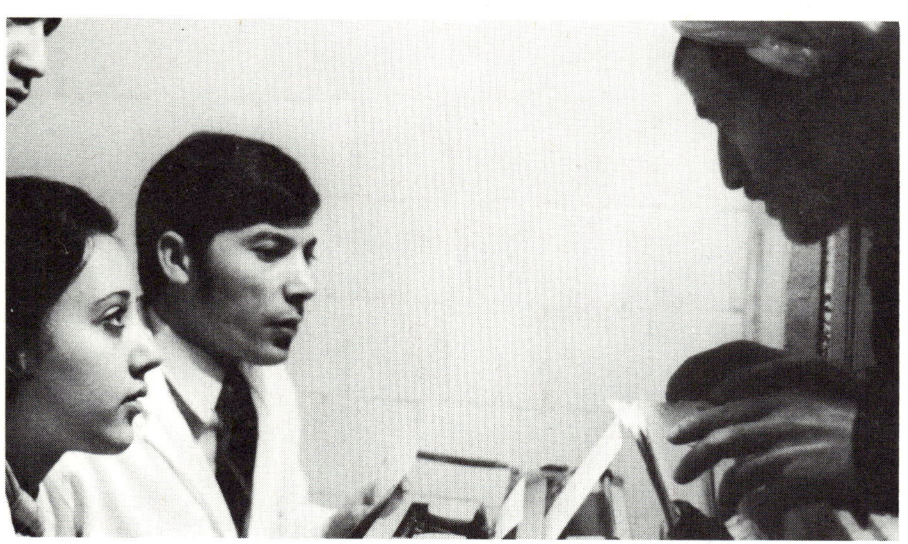

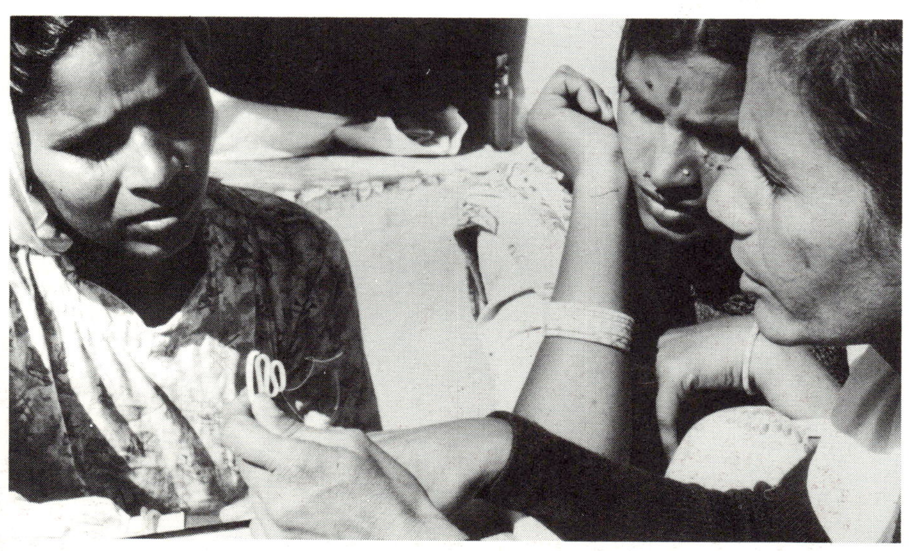

In Iran, a study
has been made
to compare
diagnostic and
therapeutic
efficacy of a
medical doctor
and an auxiliary.
There was
surprisingly
little difference
between the two.

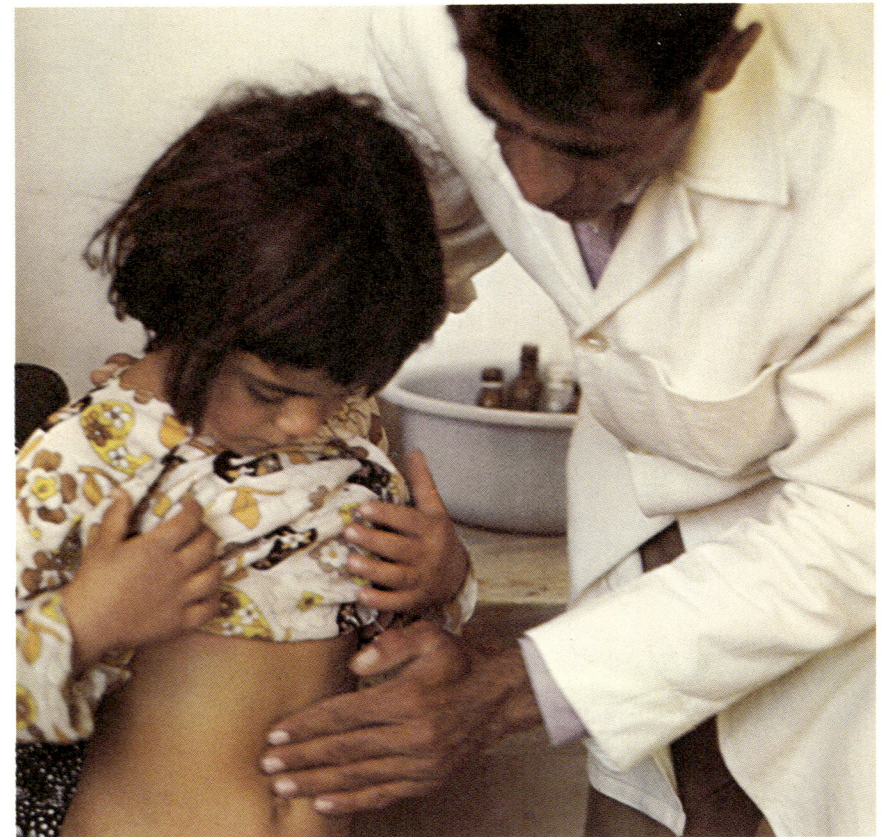

Several pilot
projects have
been carried out
to provide
health care
delivery to
isolated villages.
A nationwide
program is now
underway to
extend the
system
throughout Iran.

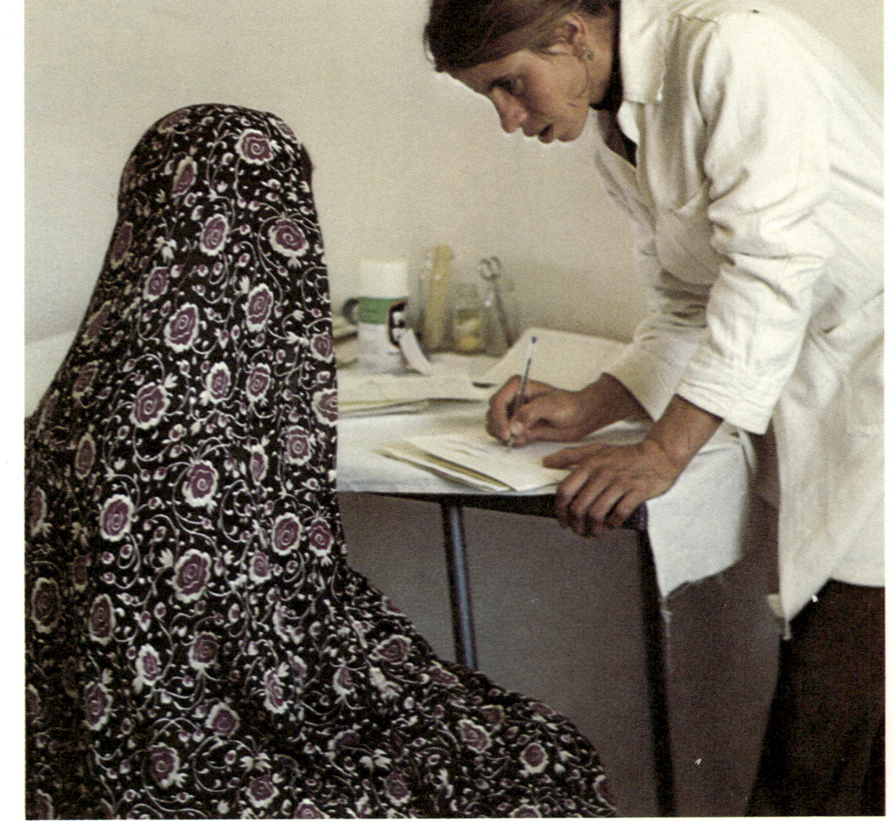

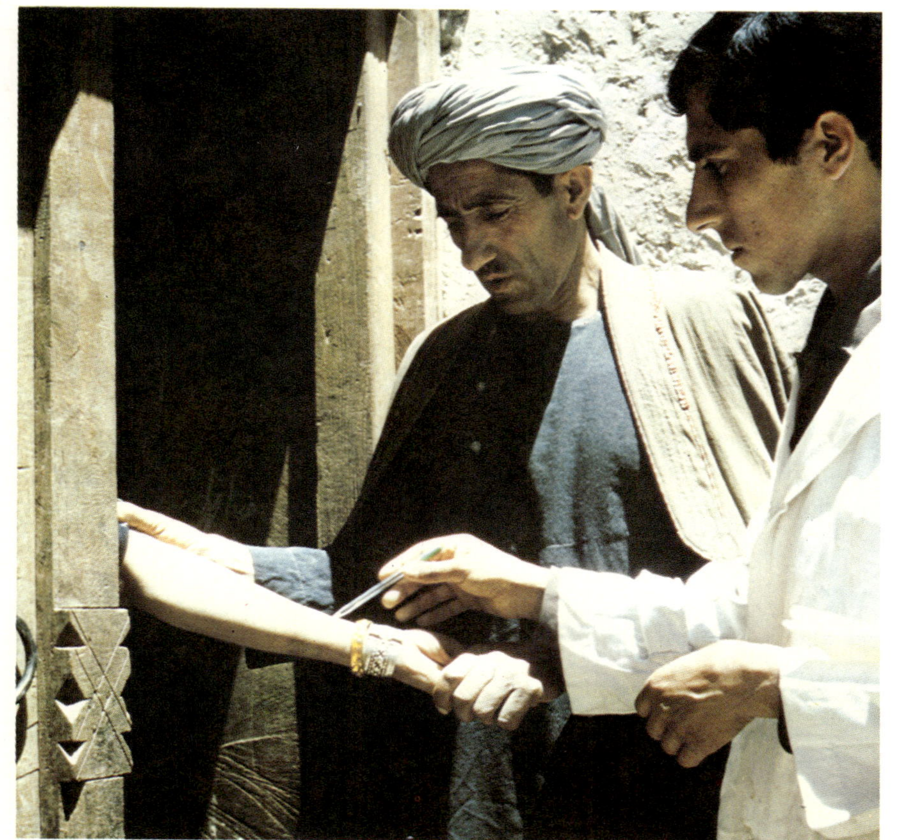

In Afghanistan, healer-training programs have also been undertaken. Here, a young doctor gives explanations to a village health worker.

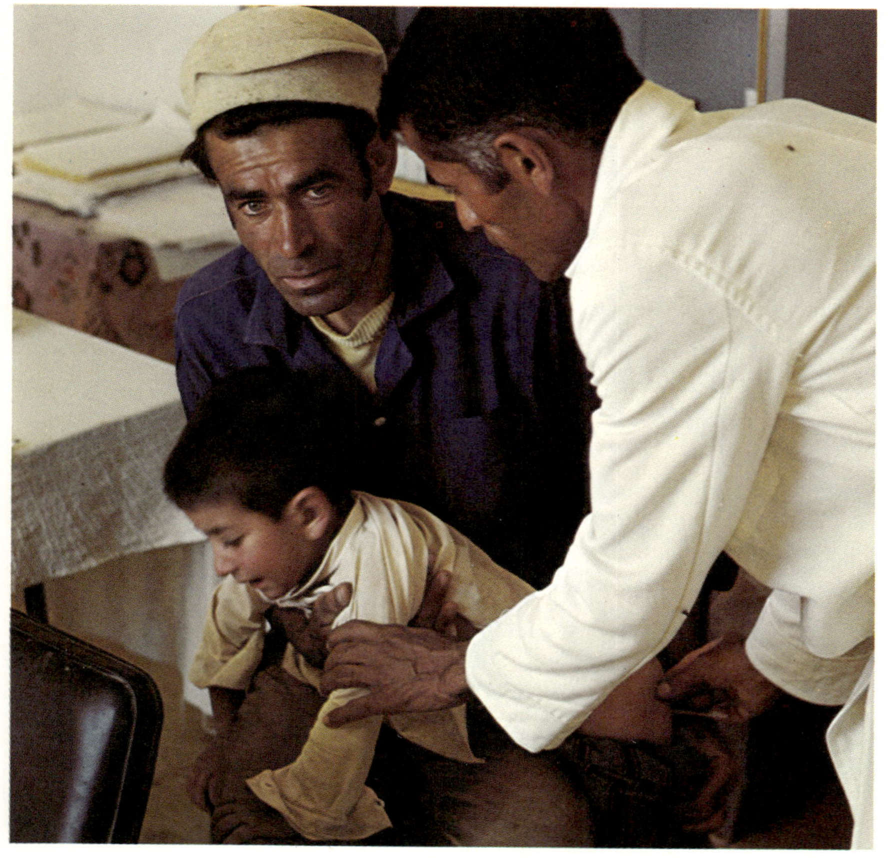

In many villages isolation and difficult access make it impossible for medical doctors to make regular rounds. Health care delivery becomes the responsibility of a trained villager.

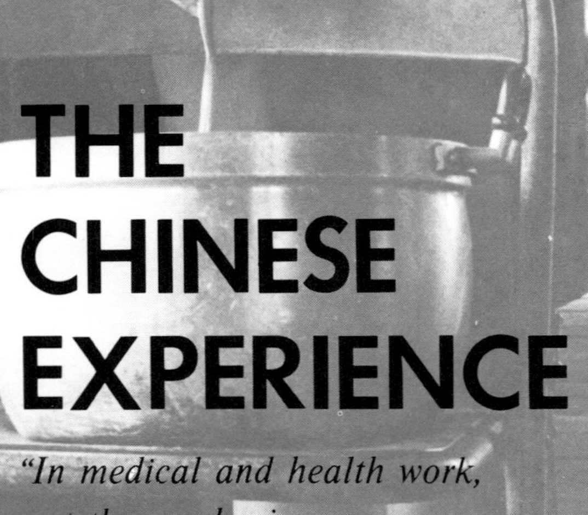

THE CHINESE EXPERIENCE

*"In medical and health work,
put the emphasis
 on the rural areas."*
Mao Tse-tung

THE CHINESE EXPERIENCE

To most Western observers, the events that have led to a complete upheaval and reorganization of the health care delivery system in China are as mysterious as the East. The results, admittedly, are amazing. In a few years, a "developing" country, cutoff from Western civilization, has singlehandedly overcome chronic malnutrition and brought under control most of the epidemic diseases that had plagued the country in the past. Child mortality has been reduced in a spectacular fashion, and something that appears to be a nationwide family planning program has been set up. In the process, the Western medical monopoly has been overturned, while many of its achievements have been incorporated into a truly national medical system, that has also benefited from the experience of countless generations of traditional practitioners.

Needless to say, China is a very particular case.

China was a semi-colonial, semi-feudal country, long subjected to outside influence and foreign aggression. In the 19th century, it was to some extent Europeanized. In large cities, the European-style medical system became prevalent, and the Chinese Medical Journal was printed in English. The pattern is only too well known. According to Dr. Chu, of the Ministry of Health, China trained about 9 000 physicians from 1927 to 1929, and some 140 000 allied medical workers.

After the success of the Chinese revolution in 1949, changes in the health care delivery system slowly gathered momentum. A first step was the introduction, in the fifties, of the teaching and practice of traditional Chinese medicine (acupuncture, moxibustion – the cauterization by burning herbs on the skin – and herbal medicine) alongside Western medicine. By 1958, there were at least 13 colleges and several hundred secondary schools capable of producing thousands of graduates to join the ranks of some 500 000 existing practitioners of traditional medicine. At the same

Who is the doctor ?
In this
Chinese commune
of the
Guangdong
province, one
of the women
in the silk
spinning plant
is a barefoot
doctor. Like
other commune
members, she
is paid on
a work-point
basis, but gives
some of her time
to preventive
and therapeutic
activities,
after having
followed a
few weeks' course
given by
itinerant
medical teams.

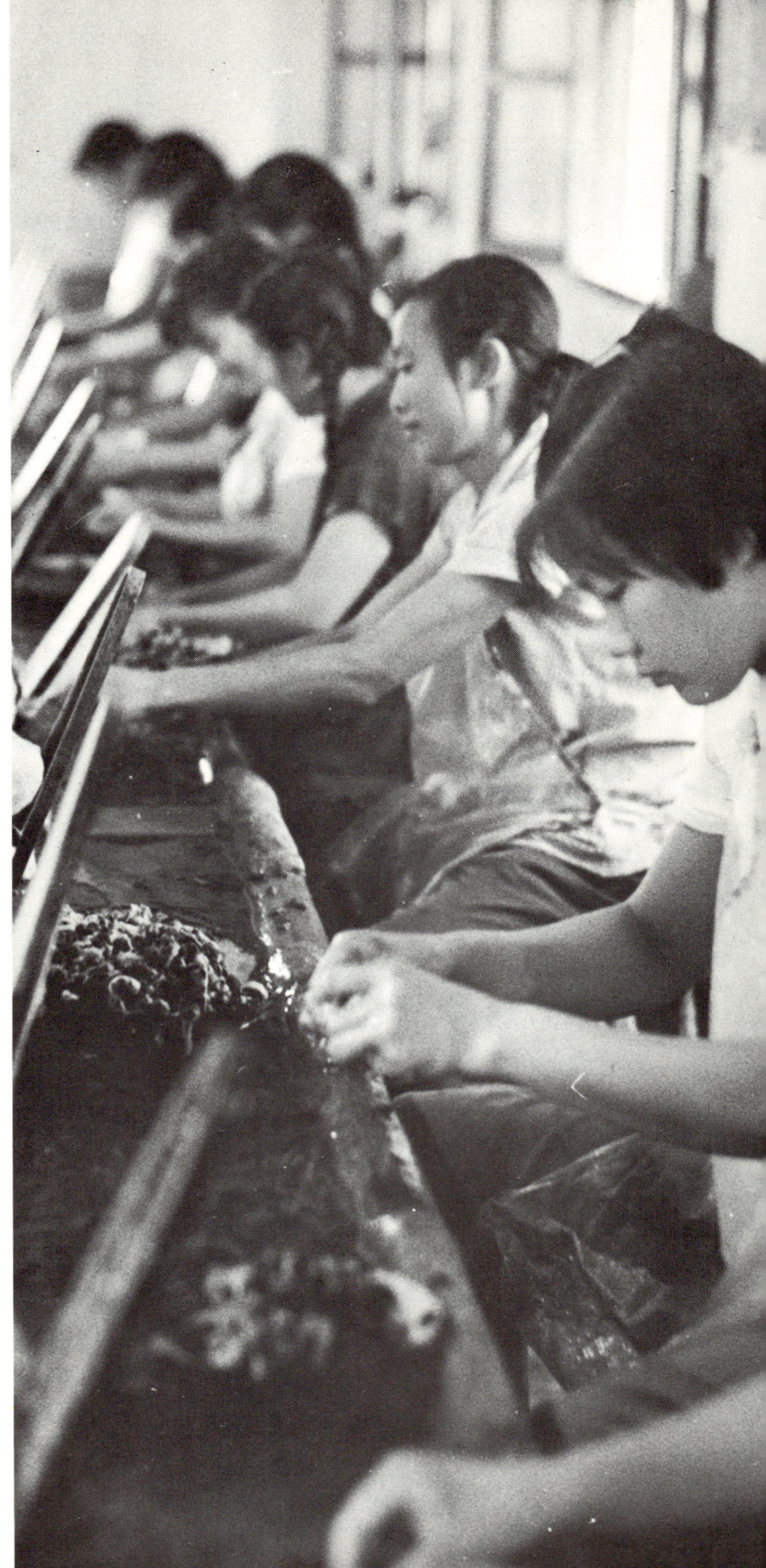

time Western-style medicine reached a high level, and the country produced its own heart-lung machines, hyperbaric oxygen operating chambers, and drugs.

But the government realized that "these so-called first class physicians ignore the existence of 500 million peasants and serve only the urban minorities." The pattern, in other words, was not so different from what it is in many former colonies.

Then, in less than a decade, the situation changed completely. In 1965, Chairman Mao asked that "in medical work, the emphasis be put on the rural areas." This was no mere aphorism, but a policy that was rapidly and effectively enforced. It gave impetus to the "barefoot doctor" system, now the backbone of health care delivery in a country of 800 million people.

The birth of barefoot doctors

It seems that the term "barefoot doctor" was first used in the Chiangchen People's Commune on the outskirts of Shanghai in 1965. This commune had one clinic with a dozen doctors and nurses to serve a population of 28 000. While treating patients, the medical team started to teach young farmers to perform some medical tasks. These peasants, like others, were paid on the basis of work-points. They continued to work in the fields, but took time to care for their fellow farmers, who affectionately called them "barefoot doctors." Barefoot doctors earn about as much as farmers, sometimes slightly more.

In the years that followed, the barefoot doctor system spread rapidly. To begin with, the government allocated more funds for medical service in the rural areas, so that most money went to where the majority of the people live. (In most developing countries, and, for that matter, industrial ones too, the reverse is true : most of the "health money" goes to the cities, where the doctors are.)

It is estimated that 700 000 doctors and medical workers joined mobile teams that travelled to remote areas, and that more than 100 000 medical graduates went to work in the countryside. Lightweight, portable equipment was developed for the mobile teams, so that even major operations could be performed in the villages, either in tents or in the homes of patients when there was no health centre.

These young doctors and the mobile medical teams started training more barefoot doctors, selected from peasants and educated young people in the countryside. The selection is generally made by commune members and approved by brigade leadership. Chosen not only for their educational background but also for their willingness to serve the people in an unselfish way, the new barefoot doctors are usually about 20 years old, and have a primary or junior high school education.

First they receive three to six months' training, either in the commune or at the county hospital, from the mobile medical teams, or in schools set up for that purpose. After a period of practice, they receive additional training and refresher courses, usually repeated at least once every year, during the slack winter season.

The training concentrates on basic medicine and treatment and prevention of the most common diseases in the area. There is no set curriculum — it is adapted to the needs, the sanitary conditions and the disease pattern in every region, and practice is integrated with theory.

Barefoot doctors learn the use of common Western drugs, of traditional medicinal herbs, acupuncture, and simple medical techniques such as injections, surgical dressing, and first aid. They practice preventive medicine and give inoculations, report communicable and seasonal diseases, organize sanitation campaigns and massive drives against rats, bedbugs, flies, mosquitoes, or snails. As a Chinese doctor, Prof. T. K. Lin, recalls it : "Each of us, regardless of whether he was a janitor or a university president, had to carry around a big fly swatter and a vengeful lust for dead flies. Everyone had his or her quota to fullfill by the end of the week."

Women barefoot doctors, in addition, become midwives, learn maternal and child care and the use of contraceptives, and perform abortions (the aspiration method is now widely used in the cities and the countryside.)

The number of barefoot doctors in China now exceeds one million. Many of them have been elected to the revolutionary committees, and the best are recommended for training in medical schools ; upon graduation, most of them return to their villages. Thus in a few years, China has managed noticeably to improve the health of a huge rural population that had been chronically ill throughout much of Chinese history. Smallpox and cholera appear to have been practically eradicated; leishmaniasis and schistosomiasis, once widespread parasitic diseases, are at least under control.

Self-reliance comes first

Throughout this "medical revolution," the emphasis was placed on two points : self-reliance, and the rural areas. During the 1974 World Health Assembly, the Chinese delegate, Prof. Huang Chia-szu stressed these points several times : "Each country should do a good job of its national health work at the basic level. As far as China is concerned, to do a good job of health work at the basic level mainly refers to health work in the rural areas." And : "The Chinese government and people have always held that only after a country has won complete independence politically and economically, can broad prospects be opened for the development of national health services."

It does not seem that the Chinese barefoot doctor system, as it has developed in its social, political and cultural background, is readily exportable as is. What is exportable, however, is the idea that non-medical healers can be of tremendous service in a country where the Western-style medical doctor does not correspond to economic or cultural realities.

It may be a hundred times less costly to train a healer, auxiliary, or barefoot doctor than it is to train a medical graduate. If the medical doctor leaves his country or remains in the city to compete with other medical doctors, while the health worker remains where he is needed, the cost accounting of health care delivery becomes overwhelmingly favourable to the health worker. And if a medical doctor can supervise, and collaborate with, health workers strategically spread out through a large area, his effectiveness is considerably increased ●

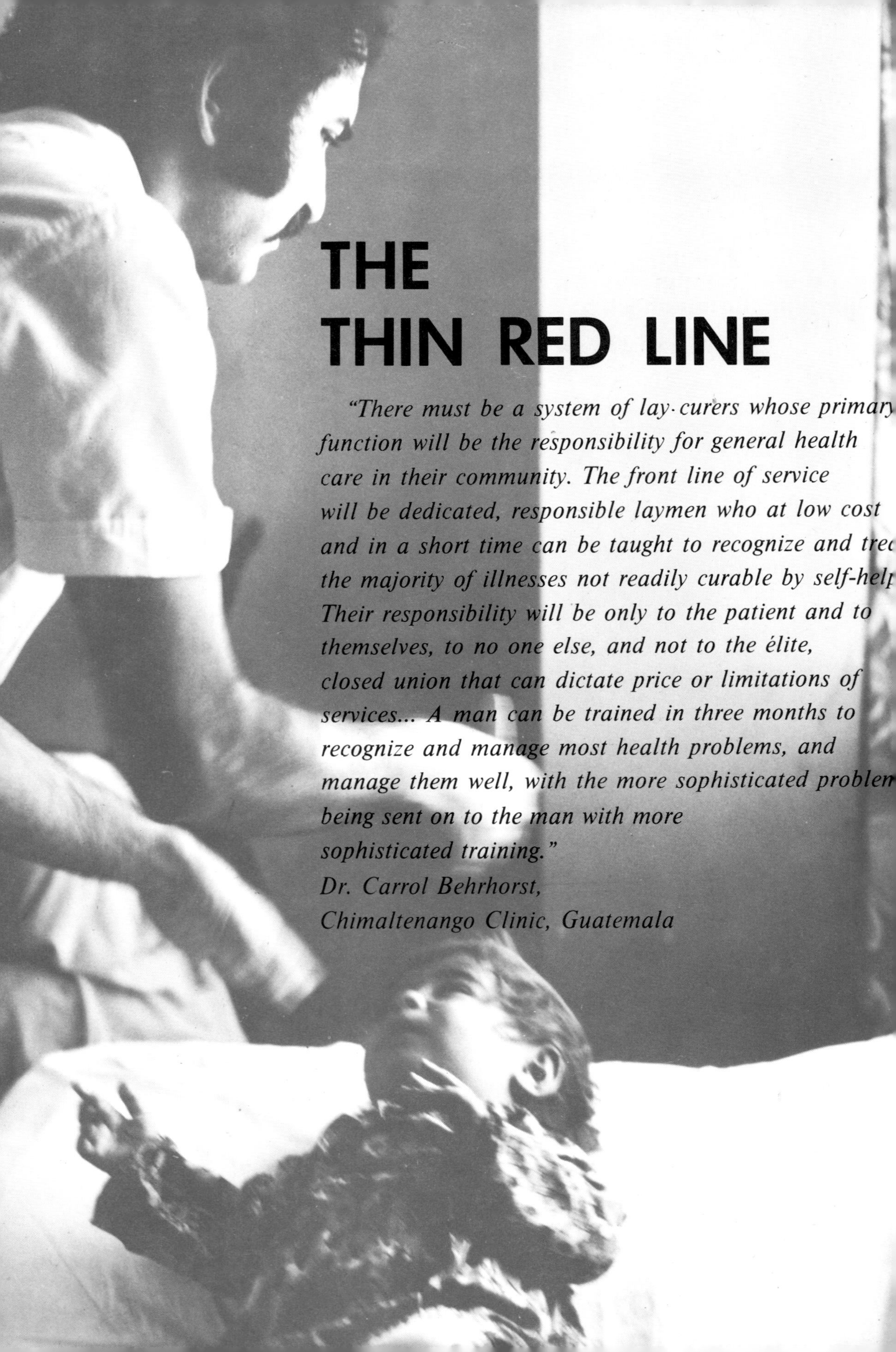

THE
THIN RED LINE
"There must be a system of lay-curers whose primary function will be the responsibility for general health care in their community. The front line of service will be dedicated, responsible laymen who at low cost and in a short time can be taught to recognize and treat the majority of illnesses not readily curable by self-help. Their responsibility will be only to the patient and to themselves, to no one else, and not to the élite, closed union that can dictate price or limitations of services... A man can be trained in three months to recognize and manage most health problems, and manage them well, with the more sophisticated problems being sent on to the man with more sophisticated training."
Dr. Carrol Behrhorst,
Chimaltenango Clinic, Guatemala

THE THIN
RED
LINE

Pedro Chacach, age 35, is a Cakchikel Indian, descendent of the Mayas of pre-Colombian Central America. He is one of the best-known and most respected men in his village, San Jose Poaquil (pop 3 000) on the high plateau of Chimaltenango above Guatemala City.

In the waiting room next to his office, there are about 20 patients. Chacach is giving a penicillin injection to a young boy whose injured hand shows signs of infection. The healer's office is part of his home, a stone and mud house with a beaten earth floor. There is a wooden table covered with a white cloth, and, around him, the now traditional symbols of the modern profession of healing : stethoscope, syringes, ampules and a medicine cabinet, and a diploma hanging on the wall. The fee for services rendered — also traditional to the profession – is respected : 25 centavos (about 25 cents) for the treatment, including the injection of penicillin.

A healer to his people

Chacach is not a medical graduate. He is bilingual, speaking both his native dialect and Spanish, and he can read and write. A few years earlier, he completed a three-month course aimed at teaching him to recognize and treat the most common medical problems in his community. On the high plateau, inhabited by some 200 000 Indians, most of whom speak only one of the region's dialects, there are about 50 such healers, with the official title and diploma of "health promoter," to deliver health care in a population where, a few years ago, between one third and one half of the children died before reaching the age of five.

As years go by, it happens that a Western-type doctor, a graduate of Guatemala City's medical school, starts regular visits to the villages, or that a health center is created nearby. The health

The stethoscope, symbol of the medical profession, can be a useful tool in the hands of an auxiliary. Here, an Ethiopian "healer" listens to a patient's heartbeat.

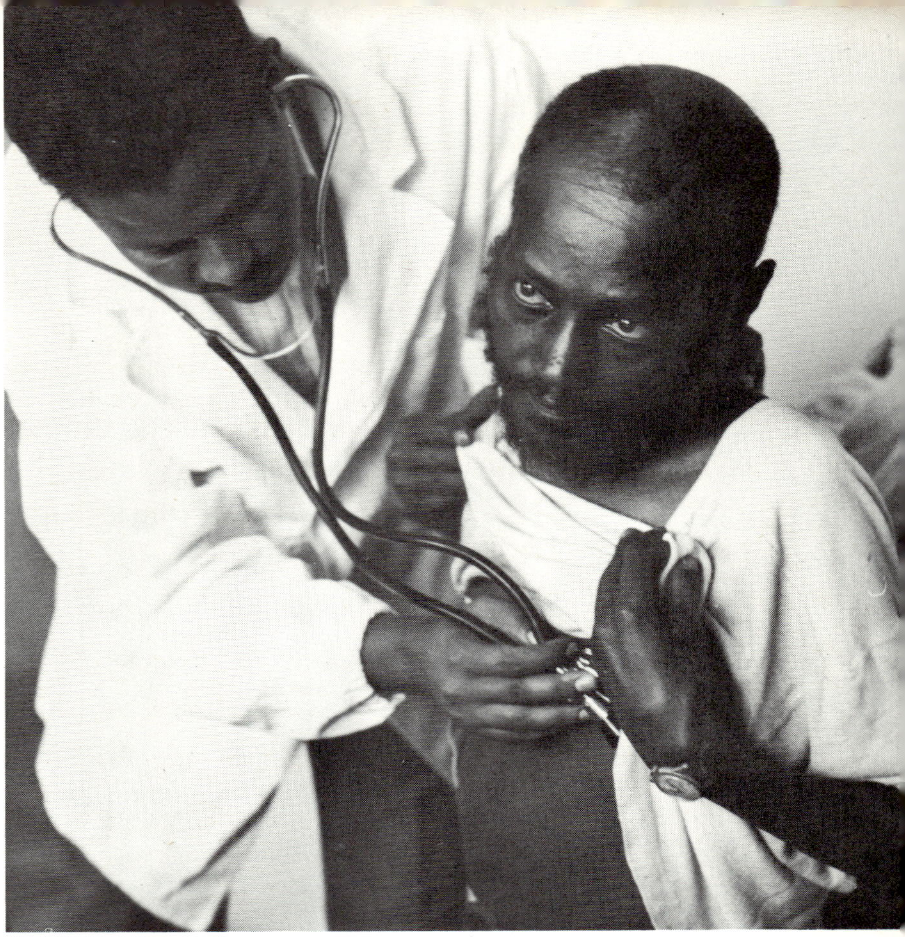

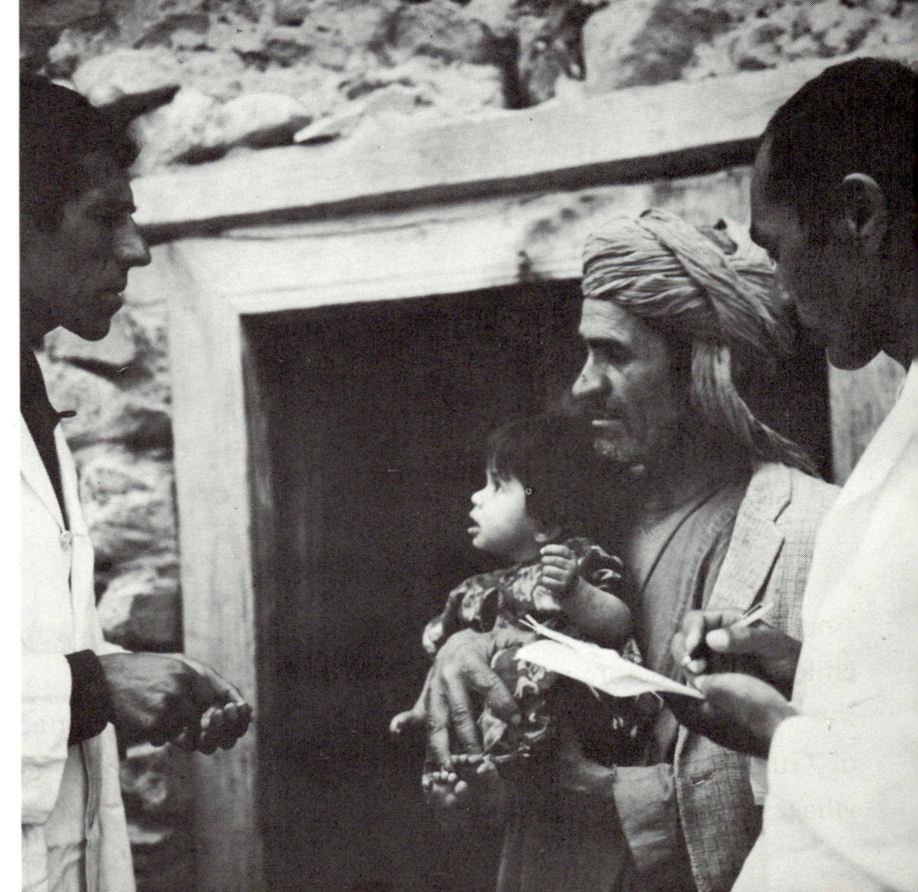

The willingness of a patient to see a healer is essential to effective health care delivery. In Afghanistan, father and son are visited by a health care team.

promoter thus finds himself in competition with the medical doctor.

Some medical doctors in Guatemala are critical of the *promo-dores* system. One of them does not hesitate to say that the system's creator, Dr. Carrol Behrhorst, should be run out of the country. It is true that Dr. Behrhorst is an American expatriate who has, with missionary zeal, set up a health system in a community of Indians he has learned to respect. The system is far from perfect. The promoter's knowledge and skill are limited, and they make errors. But would the disappearance of the system and Dr. Behrhorst's return to the United States (where he could discuss the problem with a number of expatriate Guatemalan physicians) be a better solution ?

A multi-tiered system

In Guatemala, a beautiful country that attracts many foreigners, at least ten separate health care delivery systems have been started in the rural areas. The latest has been undertaken by the Ministry of Health with the technical assistance of another American doctor, E. Croft Long. It consists of training "rural health technicians" who receive two years of medical training and will be assigned to work in rural areas as salaried ministry employees under medical supervision. They will represent an intermediary step between the health promoters and the medical doctors, part of a multi-tiered health care delivery system that will be much less costly to create and to maintain than a hypothetical coverage of the needs of the country by medical doctors, who would have to be produced, and persuaded to stay in rural areas.

A pattern adapted to the needs

Dozens of such systems are being tried throughout the world. They cannot follow a set pattern, but must be adapted to local conditions. Only one set pattern has been almost universally tried – that of the Western medical establishment ; the considerable investment has not given adequate returns.

The importance of the environment in which a health care system operates was demonstrated by Dr. Hossain Ronaghy, of

Shiraz, Iran. He has provided a selected number of villagers with medical training similar to that received by Chinese barefoot doctors ; but the result was not a crop of Iranian barefoot doctors.

"Iranians are a highly individualistic people with a limited history of cooperative enterprise, whereas the Chinese have a long history of close cooperation (such as irrigation works) made imperative by the intense crowding in the great river valleys," writes Dr. Ronaghy. Perhaps because of this, the Iranian auxiliaries *(komak behdars)* became more interested in individual, curative medicine, diagnosis and prescription of treatment, whereas the educational and sanitary aspects of the work, strongly emphasized in the teaching (and so successfully carried out in China) elicited less enthusiasm.

Multiple levels of training

If the Chinese barefoot doctor system is not exportable, the idea of a multi-tiered health personnel is, provided the tiers are adapted to the local needs. Levels of healer training can range from a few weeks to a few months, even a few years, approaching the level of the Western practitioner. Such an approach has been taken in Yaounde, Cameroon, where a six-year course leads to the formation of medical doctors who are not exportable, and who are expected to work in teams with auxiliaries and nurses. However, a few of the graduates of this new school of health sciences have expressed interest in completing their training abroad. And this, too often, is a first step towards emigration.

For there is a strong temptation to cross the thin red line that separates medical graduates from other healers, because an extraordinary prestige has been associated with those who are anointed by medical faculties and academies. The temptation of a medical doctor to go higher, into super-specialization, is not so great, because he has already crossed the line and joined the ranks of officers and gentlemen.

The existence of this "red line," or sudden discontinuity in the gradual progression of hundreds of possible levels of skill and knowledge, has created class distinctions, and helps maintain the monopoly. The social usefulness, ability, and dedication of the healer have no relevance in this distinction.

The elimination of this artificial gap and the full recognition of non-medical graduate healers may be among the most important prerequisites for the creation of an effective health care delivery system. Here is how Dr. Simon Bedaya-Ngaro, director of Public Health and Social Affairs of the Central African Republic, views the importance of the "medical assistant" as a full-fledged member of the medical team : "Recruited and trained at a level higher than that of a nurse but lower than that of a doctor, he should know how to guide and supervise the former, and to assist and relieve the latter. If necessary, he should be capable of replacing the doctor with a clear delegation of authority... He should be ready to act independently in districts where there are no doctors... By the time of his retirement, his pay and privileges should be equivalent to those of a doctor in mid career. He should know that he has a rewarding career ahead of him, and that he will be fullfilling an important role in building a better future for his country."

Iran : sweeping reforms envisaged

Such a system does not negate the role of medical doctors as essential members of the team. But when doctors are scarce, their skills should not be wasted on tasks that others can perform as well.

It is true that the reorganization of a nationwide health service, however inadequate, in the face of an established and powerful medical order, is a difficult task, almost a revolution. China has done it in relatively few years, thanks to a very particular, and perhaps unexportable, political system. Another country, Iran (which finds itself in the position of being a rich developing country) is envisaging rapid and sweeping reforms. In 1974, Prof. Anushirvan Pouyan, Minister of Health, announced that a budget had been approved for the training of 50 000 auxiliaries, to deliver front-line health care to Iran's rural population of about 20 million, scattered throughout some 55 000 villages. Two thousand auxiliaries were to be trained within a year – an impressive first step ; the auxiliaries would include nurses, assistant nurses, doctors' aides, and front-line health workers.

The plan also provided for the creation of a four-year Bachelor of Science program in health sciences, and an attempt to compress

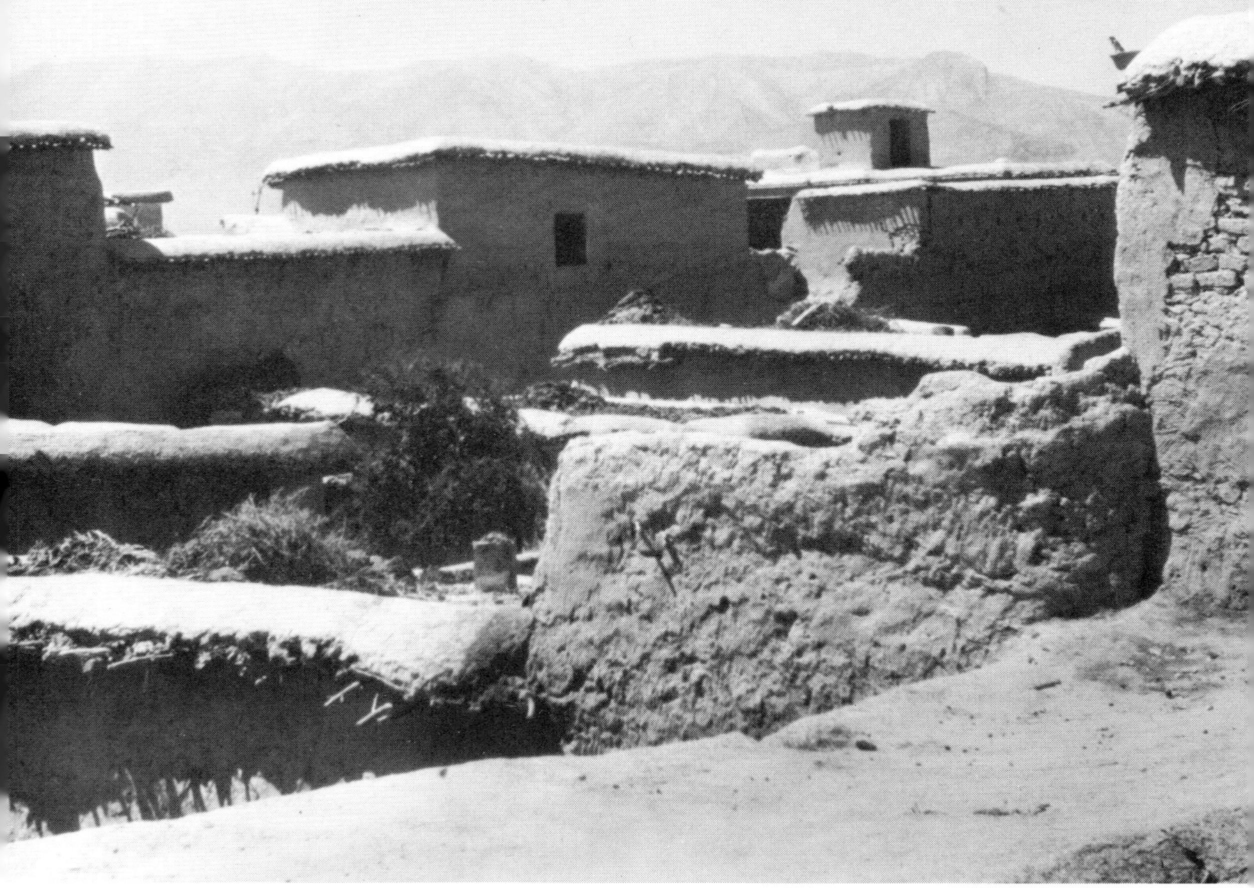

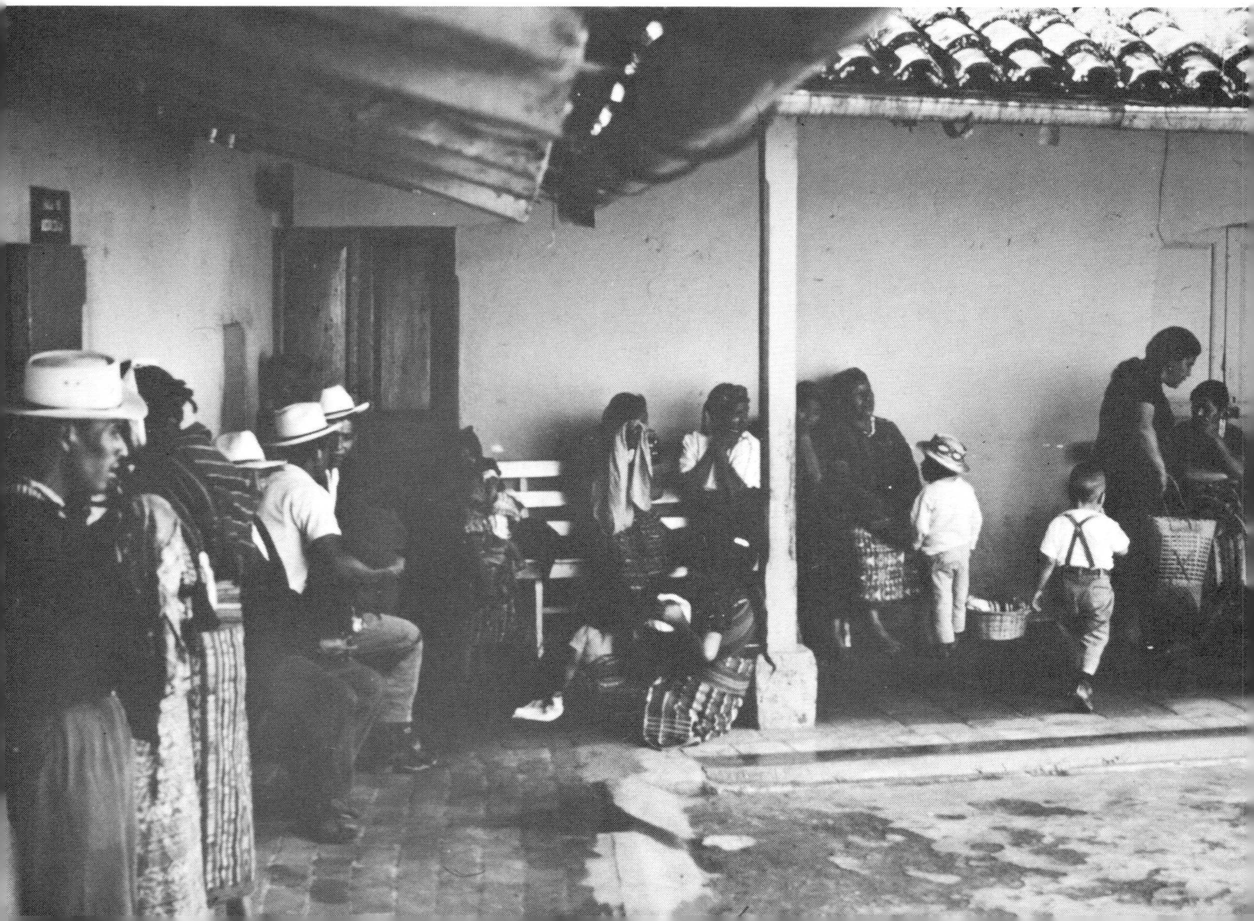